Making Miracles Happen

Making Miracles Happen

Gregory White Smith and

Steven Naifeh

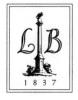

LITTLE, BROWN AND COMPANY *Boston New York Toronto London*

First Edition

Smith, Gregory White.
   Making miracles happen / Gregory White Smith and Steven Naifeh.—1st ed.
      p. cm.
   ISBN 0-316-59788-0
   1. Smith, Gregory White—Health.   2, Brain—Tumors—Patients—United States—Biography.   I. Naifeh, Steven W.   II. Title.
RC280.B7S54   1997
362. 1'9699281'0092—dc20
[B]   96-36397

10 9 8 7 6 5 4 3 2 1

MV-NY

Published simultaneously in Canada by Little, Brown & Company (Canada) Limited

Printed in the United States of America

To
Dr. Mary Lee Vance
for caring,
and caring for

Contents

Acknowledgments

My purpose is to be helpful.

Other writers have used their illnesses as raw material, as excuse, as metaphor, as memoir, as myth. But not me. My purpose in telling the story of my twenty-year ordeal with a brain tumor is only this: to be helpful. By sharing my experience, and the similar experiences of others (and the wisdom of the doctors who treat patients like us), I hope to bring some light and air into what seems — I remember well — like the darkest and most claustrophobic place on earth: the fear of dying.

My thanks to the many patients who contributed their stories, not only for giving me different perspectives on the crises and choices every patient faces, but also for teaching me humility; for showing me that, as journeys back from the edge of death go, mine has been, relatively speaking, an easy one. Telling their stories, too, makes me feel better — less self-obsessed, more *helpful* — about telling my own.

These are the real heroes of this book (both the patients and their "angels"): Charles and Doris Adkins, Richard Bloch, Michelle Webb Christian, Luana Cruz, Jeremy Eisen, Louise and Tamara

Enoch, Sara and Steven Glassner, John Grout, Ann Harrison, Andrea Hecht, Faith Hubley, Phyllis Forbes Kerr, Robert Knutzen, Rhonda Kraemer, Sean Lavery, Marilyn and Michael Leonard, Harold Lindsell, Max Marsh, Elsie Milard, Robert and Sheila Miner, Carol Ohnemus, Kim Peay, Gary Shields, Morton Silberman, Rocky Stone, Jane Taraborelli, Steven Terkel, Jacquelyn Mayer Townsend, Alice Trillin, Darren Weber, and Frances Webb. (A few patients whose ordeals are described in the book requested that I change their names when telling their stories and I have respected those requests. In the book, they are referred to as Harold and Melissa Taylor, Catherine LeDuc, Suzanne Post, and Betty Robinson.)

My thanks also to the doctors — some of the preeminent physicians in America — who contributed their remarkable intelligence, thoughtfulness, and eloquence to this book: Harold P. Adams, Richard L. Anderson, Nancy L. Ascher, Murray F. Brennan, Bruce D. Browner, Robert J. Brumback, Louis R. Caplan, Michael W. Chapman, George Panagiotis Chrousos, James Cimino, Joel D. Cooper, Jeffrey Glassroth, Hermes C. Grillo, James K. Kirklin, Samuel C. Klagsbrun, Nicholas T. Kouchoukos, W. Marston Linehan, Neil MacIntyre, Martin Miles Malawer, Rick Marder, John J. Marini, Henry Masur, J. P. Mohr, David Peretz, Thomas L. Petty, Phillip A. Pizzo, Robert S. Rigolosi, Edward C. Rosenow, Peter T. Scardino, Gordon F. Schwartz, F. John Service, Donald G. Skinner, Michael F. Sorrell, Bennett M. Stein, Mary Lee Vance, Andrew C. von Eschenbach, Dorothy A. White, William C. Wood, and Michael J. Zinner. Whatever the media may say about their profession in general, these are men and women of truly extraordinary humanity, compassion, and dedication to what is, when rightly viewed, one of humankind's highest callings: the healing arts.

A number of other people — some of them doctors, all of them caring — helped me understand better the nonmedical problems patients face. My thanks especially to Linda Anderson of the

National Cancer Institute Press Office, Virginia Andriola of the Brain Tumors Group, Marjorie Anderson of the National Stroke Association, Dr. Madelon Baranoski of Yale University, Maryanne Beratan of the National Medical Library, Diane Blum of Cancer Care, Inc., Pat Farrell of the Neurological Institute of Columbia-Presbyterian Medical Center, as well as Dr. Hannah Hedrick and John H. Henning, both of the American Medical Association.

Finally, my thanks to my twenty-three-year partner and co-author, Steve Naifeh. This book may be written in the first person, but it is as much a joint effort as any of our other books. Indeed, the story that follows was not only jointly written, it was jointly lived.

G.W.S.

Making Miracles Happen

Three Months

THEY SAID I had three months to live.

According to the doctors, a benign brain tumor, which I had been managing nicely (thank you) for more than a decade, had suddenly turned malignant. After just a few months of undetected, exponential growth, it was now, suddenly, officially "inoperable."

Thus, the inevitable question (asked like a bad actor in a B movie): "How long do I have?"

Thus, the inevitable answer (delivered with studied, stunning off-handedness): "Three months. Maybe six."

That was ten years ago: December, 1986 — just a week before Christmas. I had flown to the Mayo Clinic in snow-covered Rochester, Minnesota, instead of home for the holidays. "Frosty the Snowman" and "Jingle Bell Rock" floated through the hospital corridors. I remember it all too well. The seasonal gaiety made the bleak news seem even more surreal, harder to absorb. The fact that it came from such a reputable institution made it even harder to deny.

So what was the first thing I did?

I went back to the hotel and ate every cinnamon bun in the coffee shop. Then I took stock of my life. I was thirty-four and halfway through the first really important book of my career as a writer: a biography of the artist Jackson Pollock. Strangely, I was far more distressed at the prospect of not finishing the book than at the prospect of not finishing my life, which, I figured, was also about halfway through.

No doubt, children, if I had had them, would have changed that calculus. But, as it was, the Pollock book *was* my child, and I grieved for the uncertainty of its future far more than the uncertainty of my own.

Not until sometime later that day, after more cinnamon buns, some calls to family and friends, and not a few tears shed in the dreadful loneliness of a hotel room, did I realize what a fool I was being. How stupid. The news was simply wrong. Not the part about the tumor — I had seen the scans myself and the ghostly lily pad of tumor floating in the little gray pond of my brain. No, what was wrong was the death sentence that the doctors read in those ghostly images.

Three months. They said I had *three months*. But what did that mean exactly? Was it like the expiration date on a carton of milk? Maybe, if conditions were favorable, if I didn't get left out too long or used too often, I might last a little longer ("maybe six"), but the laws of spoilage, like the laws of aging, were irreversible and inescapable? Or was it like the expiration date on a driver's license? As long as I was safe and careful, or lucky, I might go on forever?

Then it hit me. As I was medicating my depression with the tranquilizer of television, a local weatherman came on to say, with an apologetic smile, "Better break out those umbrellas, friends. Tomorrow's gonna be a wet one." In my fatalistic mood, I thought, "Oh great. Just what I need. How appropriate." The dark clouds, the shrouds of freezing rain. God was giving stage directions for

4

my last act ("thunder and lightning off stage left"). The smiling weatherman was followed by one of those playschool graphics with a frowning sun holding an umbrella and the words "Tomorrow: 90 percent chance of rain."

That was it. *My doctors were weathermen!* They were making predictions based on previous experience, not on immutable laws of nature. When the weatherman said "rain tomorrow," what he meant was "there's a good *chance* of rain tomorrow — a 90 percent chance — but still just a chance. Out of every ten days with the same or similar atmospheric conditions, it will rain on nine of them —*but not on one.* Rain is a good bet — a very good bet — *but not a sure thing.*"

In other words, it was all about *odds.* My doctors were just better-educated, better-paid weathermen making predictions about the course of my illness based on previous experience. When they said "three months," they were reading a statistical table, not a crystal ball. What they really meant was not that *I* would die in three months, but that a substantial majority of patients with symptoms like mine died within three months.

A substantial majority —*but not all.*

All I had to do was somehow find my way into that minority who slipped by the three-month expiration date — and then, maybe, the six-month one as well. All I had to do was be that one sunny day out of ten. All I had to do was beat the odds.

Like every other patient, I heard the question "Why me?" in every tentative beat of my heart. But even before that, I wanted to know "How me?" How did this happen?

For a long time, the only answer I could get from doctors was "idiopathic," which is the Greek way doctors shrug their shoulders and say, "Beats the hell out of me." Later, after plotting the tumor's growth rate and reconstructing events prior to its debut, I was able to identify what I think — although not all my doctors agree — was the "big bang," the very instant at which my universe of medical problems began.

It was 1971 and I was doing the spring vacation thing with some college buddies. We were playing around the pool of a little motel in Fort Lauderdale pretending to shoot each other and doing stunt falls into the water. On one particularly spectacular "death" off the diving board, I went straight to the bottom and hit head-first. I knew instantly I was in trouble. As I floated upward, I struggled to keep from blacking out. I kept telling myself, "Don't let go. Stay conscious. Just get to the surface." When I finally breached, I was holding my head. "I hurt myself," I called out with what seems, in retrospect, extraordinary poise. But my friends thought I was still fooling around, just *playing* wounded, so they laughed. "No, I really *am* hurt," I insisted. And just then, as if on cue, a veil of watery blood streamed out from under my hand and covered my face. "That'll teach 'em to laugh at me," I thought as they rushed me to the hospital.

Fifteen years later, I was in New York, writing the Pollock biography. Along with Steve Naifeh, my law school classmate and co-author, I was attending a Christmas party when I tried to take a sip from a glass of punch and the ruby-red liquid dribbled down my chin and onto my shirt. I started to explain, but my lips wouldn't form the *b* in trouble, or the *p* in panic. "Help" came out "Hell." And that's exactly what it was. The right side of my face was paralyzed. I couldn't even pucker to kiss the hostess a frantic goodnight as I fled the room in terror.

Just a few days later, I was in the hotel room with the cinnamon buns and the playschool graphics, thinking about expiration dates and sunny days, and hearing that doctor's voice in my head, again and again, impossibly calm: "Three months, three months, three months."

How did it feel?

That's the question I've been asked most often in the ten years since my Christmas at Mayo. How did it feel to be told I only had three months to live? How did it feel to find out suddenly that my life was going to be cut short, without warning or recourse? For years, I struggled to find a good answer to that question. I tried all the canned responses — "I was shocked / stunned / amazed / speechless," or, "It felt unreal / like a dream / like a movie / like it was happening to somebody else" — but they just never seemed adequate. Some caught the helplessness but missed the terror; others caught the dread but missed the panic.

It wasn't until recently, when Steve and I started work on this book, that I found the answer I'd been looking for: the answer to "How did it feel?" It came from a patient named Darren Weber.

In 1991, Weber was a twenty-six-year-old communications sergeant in the U.S. Army's elite Special Forces. He had been called up after four years of inactive status, during which he earned his college degree, because of the Gulf War. Before he could join Desert Storm, however, he needed a refresher course in parachute jumping. That was how he found himself in a helicopter eleven thousand feet above the Oklahoma prairie.

As a Green Beret, Weber was an old hand at military free-fall parachuting. Indeed, his first two jumps that day went without a hitch. By the third jump, his confidence was back. Finally, he could relax and enjoy the sheer exhilaration of free-falling more than six thousand feet at 120 miles per hour, through a cool, cloudless sky. He even did a few stunts in mid-air — rotation left, rotation right — before picking up the drop zone and "just flying my body toward it." Within only a few seconds, Weber had reached his "pull altitude," four thousand feet, when it was time to pull the ripcord that opened his parachute, and begin his slow descent to the ground.

Only, when he reached for his ripcord, it wasn't there.

With his body arched in free-fall position and the ground approaching at the speed of a bullet train, he felt everywhere for the ripcord. He thought maybe it had worked its way down. Nothing there. Maybe up. Nothing there. After searching for two or three seconds — the exact amount of time the army manual allowed — Weber decided to undertake what the manual called "emergency procedures." He pulled his reserve chute.

It didn't open. One of the steering lines had ripped away and wrapped around the slider, a square of nylon designed to keep the parachute from opening too quickly. The chute was deployed but catching about as much air as a garbage bag with the open end tied shut. It looked more like a streamer than an umbrella. When Weber looked up, he saw blue sky where his parachute should have been.

The manual called it a "non-inflated canopy." But Weber had his own words for it, and he shouted them into the microphone in his helmet to his horrified comrades on the ground: "All I've got is a bunch of crap."

The ground was three thousand feet away now. Still approaching at 120 miles per hour. At that rate, Weber figured, he would reach it in about fifteen seconds.

No main parachute. No reserve parachute. The manual had a term for that, too: "total malfunction."

In his helmet, Weber could hear his comrades on the ground yelling at him, "Cut away, cut away," thinking that it was his main chute that had failed to deploy and urging him to go to his reserve chute, not realizing that the garbage bag above his head *was* his reserve chute. He tried screaming into his microphone to tell them, but couldn't make himself understood.

Meanwhile, every five seconds brought the ground another thousand feet closer.

In the few seconds he had left, Weber tried to force air into the canopy by pumping the rear risers — "like putting on the brakes" — but the effort only pushed him into a corkscrew downward spiral.

At five hundred feet, he was winded, he couldn't breathe, his parachute was still a streamer, and he was plummeting toward the earth in a dizzying, hundred-mile-an-hour corkscrew, in what the manual euphemistically called "an extreme descent."

With the ground less than two seconds away, Weber "assumed the position," the impact position that he had learned in airborne school years before: "Put your feet and knees together. And relax."

Relax!

Darren Weber hit the ground at ninety miles an hour. Only he didn't hit the ground. He hit the asphalt runway.

That's how it feels.

That's the way I felt when the doctor told me I had three months to live. Not the hitting part (although there was a momentary breathlessness, as if I'd been sucker-punched in the stomach); but the *falling* part — the feeling not just of helplessness, but of frantic, silent helplessness; the sense of disconnection from the world, from everything familiar and secure, the vast aloneness; the sense of events rushing by in a blur of futility, of time accelerating just when you need it most to slow down; the terror of hurtling toward an end every bit as abrupt and unavoidable as the Oklahoma earth, pulled by a force as inexorable and implacable as gravity. *That's* how it feels to be told you have a life-threatening illness. And I know from talking to other patients that the feeling is the same whether the doctor says "brain tumor" or "breast cancer" or "prostate cancer" or "emphysema" or "AIDS" or any one of a thousand rarer catastrophes. Every one is a push out of the plane.

What else does the case of a writer with an inoperable brain tumor have in common with that of a Special Forces sergeant who fell from eleven thousand feet onto an airport runway?

For one thing, we both lived.

The same helicopter from which Weber jumped rushed him to a nearby hospital and within ten minutes he was in the emergency room. His right arm and both his legs were broken. One leg was "externally rotated" — the foot pointed out to the side. The other leg, the one he landed on, had been pushed into his pelvis, making it an inch and a half shorter than the other. His back was broken in four places, his pelvis in three, his ribs in two. Internally, he had bruised his lungs and torn his liver. At one point, his lungs filled up with fluid and he stopped breathingaltogether.

Five years and six surgeries later, Darren Weber is still walking. And ten years after that bleak Christmas, I'm still writing.

In fact, my story and Darren Weber's have a lot in common. And our stories, in turn, have a lot in common with the stories of the other patients I spoke to for this book: patients who survived catastrophic medical ordeals when nobody thought they would; patients whose backgrounds and diseases differ as much as mine and Darren Weber's — from a ninety-year-old oil worker with kidney failure to an eight-year-old schoolgirl with bone cancer, from an international banker with malignant melanoma to a grocery clerk with cystic fibrosis, from a ballet dancer with a spinal tumor to a weightlifter with a cerebral hemorrhage, from a former nun with breast cancer to a former Miss America with a massive stroke.

Like all these patients, Darren Weber found his way to the best medical care available. The Army fixed some things, but "washed their hands" of his shortened leg and the limp it caused. Fortunately, Weber ended up in the extraordinary hands of Dr. Michael Chapman of the University of California, Davis, Medical Center, one of the leading orthopedic surgeons in the world. It's because of Chapman that Darren Weber can walk, jog, even play basketball again, with only the trace of a limp.

Like all these patients, Weber brought to his long ordeal a determination to survive. "I had an attitude that I would never give up no matter what," he says. "If one avenue of approach seemed to close for me, I would look for a different angle. I was always asking myself, 'What else can I do?'"

Like all these patients, Weber did not have to face his ordeal alone. His entire family flew from New Jersey to Oklahoma within two days of the accident. "That meant a lot to me," he recalls.

There is one thing, however, that all these patients had that Darren Weber did not have; something that trauma patients like Weber rarely have; something, indeed, that most patients don't know they have or think they've lost when, in fact, they haven't. And it's something that can make the difference between life and death.

Control.

TWO

Taking Control

LIKE A LOT of baby boomers, I always thought I was in control. My life was *my* life. My parents, as students of Dr. Spock, believed in letting me make my own decisions from an early age. When I graduated from fourth grade, they gave me a choice between some home gym equipment (which, in the fifties, meant a punching bag and some barbells) or a trip to summer camp. To my everlasting regret, I chose camp. But at least it was my choice. By the time I was twelve, I had a forty-hour-a-week summer job as a dishwasher (albeit in my father's restaurant), and with my earnings bought my own clothes and paid all my expenses for the school year.

As a high school senior in Columbus, Ohio, I picked my college and, at age seventeen, headed east to start a new life where I would be completely in control (it was, after all, the late sixties by now). As a college senior, I picked my career: law; and my school: Harvard Law. In law school, I picked my life partner, Steve. Then, finally, after graduating from law school, I picked my career: writing. This, I thought, was the ultimate act of control: to choose *not* to be a lawyer; to reject the enticements of big law firms, the encouragement of family, and the lure of security for the creative uncertainty of the literary life.

Sure, some of my early efforts —*Moving Up in Style, Why Can't Men Open Up?*— were not exactly the literary masterpieces I aspired to write, but they paid the rent and laid the groundwork. And at least I was pursuing the career path *I* had chosen. Only the very rich and the very callous have the kind of control over their lives that permits them to do always and only what they want. By most people's standards, and certainly by my own, I was in control of my life. The decision to do the Pollock biography was proof of that. Only someone who had his life completely under control could devote ten years to a book with so little chance of commercial success.

Then came that awful Christmas. In a novelistic touch, the party where the punch dribbled from my mouth and I couldn't kiss the hostess goodnight was given by the editor of the Pollock book, Carol Southern. Perfect: total loss of control at a celebration for the *pièce de résistance* of my control.

And I do mean total. I couldn't even control my smile. I had to pinch one side of my mouth closed to drink from a straw. I had to tape my eyelid shut at night. I couldn't whistle. Without the benefit of explosive consonants, I had to struggle to make myself understood even in the simplest ways: ordering a meal, buying a plane ticket, making an appointment. It was as if I had been struck suddenly dumb — only worse. A mute could point to his open mouth and shrug disarmingly. People might think he just had a bad case of laryngitis. Deprived only of a few consonants, I would get a running start on a sentence, only to have it jump the tracks and crash into incoherence at the first *p* or *b*.

Not only had I lost control of my mouth and my face, but of what was behind it, too. Growing somewhere behind my eye was a mass I couldn't see, in a place no surgeon could reach. And it had brought with it into my life a group of strangers in white coats who were telling me how much longer I had to live, and what I *had* to do in the little time left to me. I hadn't just lost control of my body, I'd lost control of my life.

When I finally arrived at my parents' home in Columbus late on Christmas Eve (without my bags; the airline had lost them), the illusion of control had completely collapsed. My parents and sister did their best to sustain the illusion, pretending to understand my mumblings and struggling not to avert their eyes from the sight of my half-melted face. They insisted that I join them on the usual round of Christmas parties — as if nothing had happened — but the charade couldn't hold up in company. After the first one, my mother saw the humiliation I felt and decided to cancel the rest. "We'll just have a family Christmas," she said, summoning up all the great powers of maternity to transform fear into compassion. We hardly talked about it at all. We didn't have to. Just decorating the tree was a colloquy of worry. Was this the last Christmas I would spend with my family? Would I ever be able to blow out a Christmas candle again or form the words to a carol? Everything I saw, it seemed, everything I did — from wrapping presents to eating snow — turned back on me as a question about the future, a question I couldn't answer.

That sense of losing control, I know now, is typical of patients who are diagnosed with life-threatening illnesses. Whether they lose control of their speech, as I did, or their sight, their limbs or their lungs, their breasts or their bladder — the feeling is the same: the feeling of being caught by ineffable forces in inexorable processes — of having your life yanked out from under you. People describe it in different ways — "powerless," "fragile," "vulnerable" — but it comes down to this: Suddenly, the one thing you thought you had complete dominion over, your body, is in open revolt; and the one thing most important to you, your future, is in somebody else's hands. No wonder people suddenly see their lives as well as their bodies spinning out of control.

14

And then, to make matters worse, at the very moment when they feel their normal, everyday life coming apart, where do people go? Where do they find themselves spending most, if not all of their time? In a *hospital!* It's hard to imagine a place (except, perhaps, for prison, which I only know by report) better designed to make one feel powerless and patronized. During my stay at Mayo, I had an angiogram, a diagnostic procedure in which a catheter is inserted in an artery and threaded toward the tumor, dye is injected through the catheter, and x-rays are snapped, giving the doctors a picture of the blood vessels feeding the tumor. Because you're strapped to a table and can't move, but are still conscious, it's a tedious, uncomfortable, and long procedure — usually about two hours. Mine lasted six. By the time it was over, I was ready to climb the walls — but, of course, I couldn't because I was strapped to the gurney. If I even stood up, I would reopen the artery where the catheter had been inserted, and that would really be a mess. So they called "transportation" to come get me, rolled me into the hall, patted me on the head, and disappeared. An hour later, I was still waiting, only now I was shivering from the cold (hospitals are air-conditioned like meat lockers, even in Minnesota, even in the winter), and desperate for a bathroom (the dye they use for angiograms goes straight to the kidneys and thence like a tide to the bladder). I couldn't move — I didn't dare — and I couldn't get anyone to move me (the only person who wandered by said she wasn't authorized to move me but promised to find me a blanket; I never saw her again). In my ignominious agony, I kept wondering, What am I doing here? How do I get out? Will I get out? Just days before, I had been in my apartment in New York working on Jackson Pollock's life. Now look at me: half-naked and shivering alone in a hospital corridor. Me with my college education, my Shakespeare and Melville, my law degree. What good did they do me now? I couldn't even control my bladder! Was this what my life had come to?

In fact, it didn't even feel like *my* life any longer. It felt as if it were happening to somebody else. I think that's why so many people say the experience of being diagnosed with a life-threatening illness is like watching a movie. They go from doctor's office to doctor's office, from tearful heart-to-hearts with family and friends to grim prehospital preparations, like sleepwalkers: partly in shock, partly in denial, and partly in a dissociated, dreamlike trance — "This isn't happening to me. This kind of thing doesn't happen to me. It happens to other people. It happens in movies."

I had that feeling for months after being diagnosed. Every time someone asked me about my "problem," I would mouth the words, "I have a brain tumor," but the words never made sense to me. The "I" and the "brain tumor" repelled each other like the like poles of a magnet. My mind refused to register them together in the same sentence. Just as it refused to register the sympathy that they inevitably elicited. To do either was to open up a black hole through which my whole life threatened to fall.

Now I know it doesn't have to be that way.

I talked to a nurse who had served in an army hospital in Vietnam during the war. Madelon Baranoski, now a professor of psychology at Yale University, saw her share of both horrific injuries and "miraculous" recoveries while in service, and the more she saw, the more she wondered: Why did some men live while others didn't? Again and again, soldiers would come in with the most mortal wounds imaginable, but still holding themselves together, relaying information from the latest firefight, making sure their families were contacted, asking about the status of their units. "As badly wounded as they were," Baranoski recalls, "they were still very much in control of their lives."

By the time they returned from the emergency room to be prepared for evacuation, however, all that had changed.

Baranoski remembers one man in particular, a sergeant, who had stepped on a mine and was brought in, almost literally, in pieces: one leg missing, the other hanging by shreds, both arms badly mangled. But he was still conscious and still giving orders. He was *in charge*. He demanded to know how his men were doing and kept asking for an intelligence officer so he could pass along important information on the enemy's position and strength.

The doctors took off both his arms and his one remaining leg. When he had stabilized, Baranoski prepared him for air evacuation to Japan.

She learned later that he died the day he arrived there.

Why? Baranoski wondered. Not, why did he die? — cause of death was usually easy to pinpoint in war. The question that haunted her was why *then*? He was well over the worst trauma: medically speaking, out of the danger zone. He could have lived. He *should* have lived. His was such an "inessential" death. If he was going to die, why not earlier — in the field, on the operating table, in transit — when Death's breath was hot on his neck? Why, after so many close brushes, at the very threshhold of recovery, did he finally succumb?

Even after she returned from Vietnam, went to graduate school in psychology, and took a job in academic medicine, Baranoski couldn't get those questions out of her head. She couldn't stop thinking about those young men like the sergeant, who came in with their bodies broken but their wills intact, then left, often only a few days later, the other way around — bodies mended, wills broken —*prepared* to die. Was it just denial? Were they just on "automatic pilot"? Or was something happening during their hospitalization to make that life-and-death change?

Determined to find the answer, Baranoski designed an experiment using three groups of rats. The first group was given electric shocks at random intervals; the second group was given shocks, too, but was also taught a way to control the shocks. The third group was given no shocks at all.

Then all the rats were injected with cancer cells.

The results startled even Baranoski. Among the rats that were given random, *uncontrollable* shocks, the death rate was 75 to 80 percent. Among the group that was able to control the shocks, on the other hand, the rate was only 25 percent. Like those wounded soldiers in Vietnam who haunted her, the rats in the first group had "learned helplessness," she concluded. "They had learned that, finally, nothing they could do would make a difference any longer. So the struggle was depleted."

It was all about control. Take away a patient's sense of control over his life, and you have hurt him more than any injury or disease. Give him back that sense of control — and you have helped him more than any drug or therapy. He can make miracles happen.

In the years since 1969, when Baranoski conducted her experiments, other researchers at other institutions have confirmed her conclusions: Patients who take control of their lives, patients who *keep* control of their lives, patients who fight the urge to surrender their fates to strangers in white lab coats, those are the patients who stand the best chance of beating the odds.

Consider the extraordinary case of an extraordinary woman, Merle Barstow, a fading Broadway actress who buried three husbands before learning in 1969 that she had advanced breast cancer. Actually, she learned about it long before she did anything about it. Fearing (probably rightly) that directors would not let her audition if they knew she was being treated for breast cancer, Merle virtually ignored the lump in her breast until it "practically popped through the skin in a massive way," to quote the doctor who treated her.

But by that time it was too late. Her first doctor, a breast surgeon, told her there was nothing he could do, although she was welcome to try chemotherapy "just in case." Merle accepted the surgeon's advice, but not his resignation. After beginning chemotherapy, she looked around for a forum in which she could talk to other patients about the trials and anxieties of cancer therapy. "The best way to beat this thing," she told her doctor, "is to get together with other women and talk about it, take hold of my life, get some control back."

To her astonishment, there was no such group to join. This was, after all, the 1960s, and support groups were still a relatively new phenomenon. So what did she do? She started her own. "What she did was outrageous," recalls Dr. Samuel Klagsbrun, a young attending psychiatrist at New York's St. Luke's hospital at the time, whom Merle recruited in her fight. "She haunted the corridors of Sinai, St. Luke's, Columbia, all the oncology clinics, just going up to women and saying, 'You're coming with me.' Within two or three weeks, she had a group of eight women, and she had created, literally, twenty-five years ago, the first cancer support group."

In a one-woman revue of theatrical anecdotes and droll, self-deprecating humor, Merle exhorted her fellow patients not to surrender control of their lives to their illness. "Thanks to these," she would say, hoisting her breasts in the air with both hands, "the clock is ticking much faster than we expected. And with only a limited amount of time left in our lives, the question is how we want to live those years or months or weeks or days or whatever we have left. Do we want to take charge of fundamental things in our lives, or are we going to just lie there and take it?"

Merle took charge of her own life with a vengeance. Fed up with the self-defeating round of fruitless auditions — she hadn't had a callback in more than a year — she vowed to give up acting and instead pursue her other great love in life: jewelry. Armed only with her newfound determination and her irresistible, Auntie Mame–ish charm, she descended on 47th Street and persuaded an antique-jewelry-dealer friend to give her $30,000 worth of gold jewelry to sell on consignment. Next, she bought a bridge table and a folding chair and opened a small booth at a flea market in New Jersey. In that first weekend she made more money than she had in an entire year as an unemployed actress. A few more weeks and she had sold all $30,000 worth and gone back for more. Before long, she was a successful businesswoman, selling antique jewelry at flea markets all over the East Coast. At the weekly support group meetings, which she never missed, she described herself as "hysterically happy."

Eighteen months later, her cancer had completely disappeared. In less than two years, Merle had gone from advanced breast cancer with ancillary nodes to absolutely clear x-rays. Dr. Klagsbrun remembers the call from her startled, incredulous oncologist. "'I don't know what you're doing, and I don't know what I'm doing,' he told Klagsbrun, 'but, boy, we'd better continue.'"

In the years since he met Merle, in the hundreds of cancer support groups he's conducted since that first one, Klagsbrun has learned that Merle's oncologist had it all wrong. It wasn't anything he was doing or, indeed, that Klagsbrun was doing. It was what *Merle* was doing that made the difference. "Those people who use the shock of cancer to take a look at the quality of their lives and make decisions about improving the quality of their lives," says Klagsbrun, "whether they succeed in actually doing so or not, whether they achieve their goals or not, *just simply the fact that they're acting on their own behalf and making decisions, attempting to shape their own lives* — those people have, in our experience, been the ones who prolong their lives and surprise their oncologists; the ones who beat the system."

But how is it possible to take control of your life at the very moment when that control has been snatched away from you? When some stranger in a white coat has ripped your life loose from its moorings and sent it spinning in directions that you can't imagine — are, in fact, terrified to imagine? When, as Virginia Andriola, the leader of a brain tumor support group, says, "the illness just comes and takes control over your life, becomes the center of your life, the focus of everything you do, the sun around which your whole world revolves." How can you take control of your life when it feels as though not only your control, but your life itself, has been stolen from you by the news, delivered in maddeningly matter-of-fact medicalese, that you have only three months to live?

At that point, the only way to take back control of your life is to take control of your illness.

I wish I could say that I figured that out on my own. It would make a better story if I could claim that when I heard the devastating news at Mayo, I immediately sprang into Merle-like action, calling doctors, reading medical texts, exploring alternative therapies, forming support groups, grilling my doctors, etc., etc. But, like most patients, I was too stunned for any of that. After emptying the coffee shop of cinnamon buns, it took all my emotional energy to call home and deliver the terrible news to my parents (leaving out the part about "three months"). Like most patients, I told myself I was at a good hospital, my doctors were competent, the scans were clear, the diagnosis unequivocal; what was the point? Why bother rehearsing that awkward, surreal scene ("I'm afraid I have bad news, Mr. Smith") with other doctors at other hospitals? Even *one* more doctor at *one* more hospital! I just wanted to get on with "whatever was next" — the most life-affirming concept I could think of. Like most patients, I surrendered to the inevitability of it all. "Whatever you say, doc. I'm all yours."

And then I met Charles Grodin.

Yes, *that* Charles Grodin, the actor/writer/TV guest and host. We were both guests at a dinner party hosted by my only celebrity friends, Phil Donahue and Marlo Thomas. Back in the mid-eighties, Steve and I had helped write the companion book to "The Human Animal," a five-hour miniseries on NBC that Phil conceived and hosted. Phil was so pleased with the results of our labors that he invited me out to Los Angeles to help write the series. My first day there, after reviewing videotapes of the work in progress, Phil asked me to drive him back to his hotel. I, of course, was starstruck, especially when strangers on the street waved and shouted, "Hey, Phil," at every stoplight. But when he fixed me with those blue eyes and asked me what I thought of the videotapes I had seen, I had to tell him the truth. "I think they could be a lot better," I said.

From then on, we were friends.

Phil and Marlo both showed great concern when they learned of my news from Mayo and, in retrospect, I wonder if they knew exactly what they were doing when they sat me next to Chuck Grodin at the dinner table that night. Perhaps Phil had briefed him in advance, or perhaps Chuck just noticed my facial paralysis — it was all I noticed — but it wasn't long before we were talking about doctors and illness — which was all I thought about. The subject was on Chuck's mind because he had just lost his ex-wife ("but dear friend") after a terrible battle with cancer.

Indeed, he talked about it like a war. They had fought for better treatment, fought for more options, fought for better therapies, fought for experimental protocols. They had been to what seemed like a hundred doctors, from small private clinics to public megahospitals, from prestigious names to backwater unknowns, from Boston to Los Angeles. "My doctor list is longer than my enemies list," I remember him saying, "although there is some overlap." He told me about his ex-wife's long struggle —*their* long struggle — to find the best care. "You've got to keep pushing and pushing for the right treatment," he said when I told him I had only been to Mayo. "You can't take what any doctor says necessarily as the last answer, I don't care where he's from. Doctors aren't gods. You always have to press for more answers. *You have to take control!*"

His eyes began to glisten as he told me about his ex-wife's death. "The cancer eventually got her," he said, "but we at least had the satisfaction of knowing everything was considered." He wasn't sure, but he thought the struggle might even have given them an extra two or three years.

Two or three years sounded a lot better than three months.

That night, at the dinner table, I decided there was only one way to escape the death sentence I had been handed. I had to wrest control of my life back from my illness, back from this unreachable mass behind my eye that distorted my speech and contorted my face, back from the black hole of inevitability. The next day I was on the phone, struggling through the missing *p*'s and *b*'s, to develop my own list of doctors and therapies and protocols and options. At a time when I didn't want to be heard or seen because of the awkwardness and humiliation of paralysis, I forced myself onto the phone and into the offices of every doctor I could find who knew anything about brain tumors and how to fight them.

The battle for control was joined.

It would be an uphill battle, a struggle not only against my own urge to denial and surrender, but the medical profession as well: a profession designed to take control *away* from patients; a profession that infantilizes patients (even combat soldiers) with its intimidating technology and humiliating routines; a profession that speaks an impenetrable language — "oncogenic osteomalacia," "hemangiopericytoma" — with an unchallengeable, we-know-better air; a profession in which, until recently, it was considered inappropriate — and still is in some hospitals — for a patient to ask the nurse, "What was my blood pressure today?"

Dr. Michael Sorrell, a nationally recognized gastroenterologist at the University of Nebraska, told me about treating an older woman, from a previous generation, when he worked as a general practitioner in a town with a population of two thousand.

"She came in, and I said, 'What's this scar from on your belly?'"

"I don't know," she said. "Dr. X operated on me."

"Did he take out your ovaries?" Sorrell asked.

"I don't know," she repeated. "He never told me."

In 1978, when Dr. Dorothy White began working as a

pulmonary specialist at New York's Memorial Sloan-Kettering, a major cancer treatment center, there were still patients who didn't know they had cancer. Some had been treated for cancer for *ten years* without being told. Family members were at least as guilty as doctors in this conspiracy of silence. "They didn't want Mother to know she had cancer," recalls White, "even though she was coming to a cancer hospital." It was all part of a previous era in medicine, says White, an era in which "the doctor would say, 'Take these pills and go through this treatment,' or 'You're going to have an operation,' and that was the *end* of it." It was an era of paternalistic doctors who knew everything and ignorant patients who just did what they were told. It was, indeed, a simpler time — before feminism, before consumerism, before Vietnam, before Watergate — a time when institutions commanded automatic respect, and unquestioning acceptance of their authority was the mark of good citizenship.

It was also a time when many patients died what army nurse Baranoski would call "inessential deaths."

Slowly but surely, however, doctors—and patients—are changing. Among the dozens of preeminent surgeons and physicians I have spoken to over the last year, virtually every one now agrees that patients who take control of their medical treatment are more likely to defy their doctors' dire predictions. "I am a physician scientist," Dr. W. Marston Linehan, head of urologic oncology at the National Cancer Institute, told me, "and, whether or not science has proved it unequivocally, my *experience* is that the people who have it in their minds that they are going to influence the sequence of events in their own health are the ones who do the best. I am never surprised by how well those people do, and I have seen that time and time again."

For proof that medicine is moving in the right direction, just look at what has happened to cardiac care in the last few decades. There was a time in this country, not long ago, when patients with critical cardiac problems were simply revived, given prescriptions, and sent home to await the next attack. Because patients were considered mere pawns in the great chess game between doctors and the Grim Reaper, there was no effort to make them collabora- tors in their own treatment — to give them control over their medical fate. Now cardiac patients are given a whole list of things *they can do:* exercise, change their diets, adjust their work habits, reduce their stress levels, etc.

Cancer patients, like me, on the other hand, are told what the treatments are and how long they can expect to live. That's it.

I heard a story about a patient in "the old days" who had lung cancer and was a heavy smoker. One day the patient asked his doctor, "Is there anything I can do? Should I stop smoking?" To which the doctor replied, "Oh, look, it's your last bit of pleasure." Unfortunately, that's still where a lot of medicine is — especially in the treatment of cancer and other terminal illnesses. The illness is considered an independent force, beyond the patient's control.

No wonder patients feel helpless. Helplessness is what they're taught. No wonder most patients, like Nurse Baranoski's take- charge sergeant reduced to passivity, like the rats who suffered shocks with no way of controlling them, surrender so readily. So prematurely. They've been taught that they have no control, and therefore no choice.

They don't know there's another way.

THREE

A Doctor Is a Doctor Is . . .

HAROLD TAYLOR THOUGHT he was in control, too. As the founder of a spectacularly successful international securities firm in London, he was more than just the master of his fate, he was, in Tom Wolfe's memorable phrase, a Master of the Universe. Then, in November 1992, his doctor called him in for what he thought was a follow-up to a routine physical. With a look of "great alarm," the doctor told him he had advanced multiple myeloma — bone marrow cancer. When Harold asked the inevitable question, the doctor hedged. "As much as three years," he said, "or as little as three months." As Harold would soon learn, that prediction was, if anything, optimistic for this fiercely lethal disease.

Harold describes his reaction as "astonishment" followed by depression. "If somebody tells you that you are going to die," he recounts with typical British reserve, "you obviously feel sort of shocked and dismayed." His wife, Melissa, on the other hand, a Missourian by birth, was outraged. "I don't believe anybody should tell you how long they think you have to live," she says. "It really knocks the stuffing out of you."

But Harold, who had been to one year of medical school before turning to high finance, refused to surrender — either to anger or to hopelessness. The same take-charge attitude that had made him a millionaire before he turned forty, quickly kicked in. "I came from a business background," he explains, "and this represented probably the greatest dilemma that I had ever encountered. So I attacked it the same way I attack problems in business: Find the best possible people (a) to participate in helping to solve the problem and (b) to find the approach which seems to have the best chance of a successful outcome."

First, that meant "discovering" the disease. Harold tried talking to his regular doctor about it, but most of what he said — especially the scary, hopeless part — turned out to be based on antiquated information. So, with Melissa's help, he reviewed all the literature he could find on multiple myeloma. When he stumbled on something he couldn't understand, he put it in a file to ask about the next time he saw a doctor. To friends, he referred to the learning process as a "journey of discovery" for which his watchwords were "clarity," "thoroughness," and "skepticism." "We were not going to be satisfied taking somebody's word for anything," says Melissa. "That's the kind of people we are."

The next step was to find "the centers of excellence for the treatment of the disease," and it was that quest that brought the Taylors across the Atlantic Ocean to Rochester, Minnesota, to see a world-famous expert at the Mayo Clinic, an *éminence grise* in the treatment of bone marrow cancer. "There weren't that many people who really specialized in the field," recalls Melissa Taylor, "and at that point, we thought one was pretty much like another."

That was always the way I felt, too. A doctor is a doctor is a doctor. I don't know where I picked up that quaint notion. Perhaps because I, like most kids, had only one family doctor growing up, Carey Paul, who offered everything from rectal exams to acne advice (A to Z, so to speak), gave flu shots and eye exams, stitched up cuts and set broken bones. And when he found a mole he didn't like the looks of, he laid me down on the padded table in his office and performed surgery right there, right then. So, naturally, I just assumed that every doctor did everything and knew everything. Popular culture abetted this notion. Other than Dr. Paul, the only doctors I knew were the fictional kind — Casey, Kildare, and later Welby — who fixed not only bodies but hearts and souls as well, no matter what their nominal specialties.

But I think the belief that all doctors are essentially the same — equally qualified, equally knowledgeable, equally skilled — springs from a far deeper source than childhood experience or TV indoctrination. Indeed, I think we *need* to believe it. When we go to a doctor, for any reason, we want to believe that there is *a solution* to our problem, *a right answer* to our question, *a cure* for what ails us. Furthermore, we want to believe that *our* doctor, like all doctors, has that solution, that answer, that cure.

Imagine how confusing it would be if we assumed the opposite: that there was more than one "right" answer, more than one possible cure; or that maybe our doctor didn't know the answer but the doctor down the street did. How could we ever have confidence in what our doctor was telling us, in the drugs he was prescribing or the therapies he was recommending? The paranoiacs among us would always be jumping from doctor to doctor in search of a more dire prognosis; the Pollyannas, in search of a rosier one.

To avoid just that kind of crisis of confidence, the American medical establishment has worked diligently to convince us that what we want to believe is true *is* true: that all doctors are more or less interchangeable. One of the less obvious reasons for putting all doctors, even psychiatrists, through the same interminable professional training is that it heightens the impression that everyone who completes that training is equally qualified. It is still the case in most American courts that *any* doctor can testify on *any* medical question. As far as the legal system is concerned, a doctor is *presumed* to be an expert on all things medical.

There are specialists, of course (although official recognition of them was slow in coming) like the bone marrow expert the Taylors found at Mayo, but the basic principle is the same: All *specialists* are interchangeable. A gynecologist is a gynecologist is a gynecologist. A myeloma expert is a myeloma expert. Sure, one doctor may have a better bedside manner than another; one may keep you in the waiting room longer; one may have fancier offices, a more efficient staff, richer clients, higher fees, etc. But when you get right down to it, when you strip away all the cosmetic differences, one doctor is pretty much like any other doctor when it comes to the important things: knowledge, skill, intelligence.

It just isn't so.

Like a lot of patients, I learned that lesson the hard way. About two years after my accident in the pool, I started having pain in my feet. (Coming as it did at the opposite end of my body, I didn't put the two together at first.) I was in Europe studying music on a fellowship after college when I noticed that it hurt to walk. At first, I just assumed I was spending too much time on my feet. Then one day, in a park in Madrid, the woman I was traveling with challenged me to a footrace. After only a few steps, I had to drop out. I hurt all over. Not just my feet, either: my hips, my knees, my ribs, everything. I was pure pain. I felt like an old sack of aching junk rattling down the bowered paths of the Retiro.

I knew then that something was wrong — definitely, terribly wrong.

So wrong, in fact, that I immediately flew home to see, who else, Carey Paul. To my surprise, Dr. Paul scratched his head in bewilderment and sent me to an orthopedist, who scratched his head and sent me on to an even more specialized specialist, a foot and ankle doctor. After a series of x-rays and an interminable examination (inflicting, alternately, stabs of pain and fits of giggles), the foot and ankle specialist solved the mystery: I was suffering from Morton's neuroma, he announced, a growth in the foot found almost exclusively in *pregnant women!*

How was this possible? I asked, pointing out that I was neither pregnant nor female.

The doctor shrugged his shoulders. Idiopathic.

In retrospect, the most remarkable thing about this story is that *I believed him.* Had there ever been a recorded case of a man having Morton's neuroma? I didn't ask. I just took it on faith, and filled the prescription he gave me for orthopedic inserts in my shoes. After all, he was a doctor. A specialist, no less. So he must have *the* answer — however bizarre it might seem.

Only it wasn't the answer. By the time I arrived at Harvard a few months later to begin law school, I could hardly move without pain. Every time I took a step, or shook someone's hand, or sneezed, or yawned, it hurt like crazy. When I rolled over in bed, the pain woke me up. A simple cough felt like a heart attack. A doctor at the Harvard Health Services listened to my story, scratched his head in bewilderment, and sent me to an HHS orthopedist, who scratched his head and sent me on to, you guessed it, a foot and ankle doctor. After yet another series of x-rays and another interminable examination, the foot and ankle specialist informed me that my pain was due to dozens of little hairline fractures, called "metafractures," in major bones throughout my body.

But what was causing them?

Idiopathic.

The best he could do was put me on crutches to relieve the pain and offer to take a little piece of bone out of my foot (where the fractures were worst) for lab analysis. The catch: I would have to stay off my feet for several weeks — in the middle of first-year law school. I said I would get back to him.

The crutches, like the inserts, did nothing except make me feel foolish (I didn't have a cast on, so no one believed that I really needed them). Finally, in desperation, I went back to Harvard

Health Services. This time, by sheer luck, I drew a new doctor, an internist named Martin Wohl. One more time I laid out my three-year chronicle of pain and befuddled doctors. Dr. Wohl, a genial, soft-spoken Mr. Magoo figure — only with a blazing intelligence behind that high professorial forehead — listened carefully, and when I was done, suggested something none of the doctors before him — seven in all — had ever mentioned: a blood test.

That was the first of many keys that unlocked the first of many doors in this Alice-in-Wonderland journey. In medical terms, my blood was a mess. For good bone formation, the body needs both calcium (as every schoolkid knows) and, less famously, phosphorus. For some reason, I had too much of the former (which meant I ran the risk of developing stones) and too little of the latter (which meant the former could not be put to good use). My kidneys were not doing their job of maintaining a sufficient level of phosphorus in my blood to allow proper bone formation. As a result, my bones had gradually weakened ("demineralized" is the jargon) until they were so brittle that just everyday use, like walking or shaking hands, could crack them. The condition was called "osteomalacia due to chronic renal phosphate leak," or, more chillingly, "phosphate diabetes."

Why was Dr. Wohl able to see something the other doctors didn't? Why did he think to ask for a blood test (hardly an obscure procedure) when no one else did? Whatever explanations I can invent — the usual diagnostic tool for bone problems is the x-ray; x-rays don't show demineralization until it's well advanced — boil down to the same self-evident truth: All doctors are not created equal.

They don't have the same experience. Medicine is an occupation where repetition breeds quality. It may not be sufficient for quality, but it is necessary. "People are really foolish to allow themselves to be a doctor's first patient for any procedure," says Dr. John Service, a diabetes expert at the Mayo Clinic, "unless of course the procedure's never been done anywhere before." One neurosurgeon may have done five pituitary operations in ten years; another, 150. Partly, this is because smaller, regional hospitals tend to send their rare and difficult cases to larger medical centers, often academic hospitals. The result is an uneven distribution of experience. Dr. Hermes Grillo, chief of thoracic surgery at the Massachusetts General Hospital, and perhaps the leading tracheal surgeon in the world, explains, "If every little hospital in the country is trying to deal *de novo* with the rare cases, there is no way they have the time, energy, or funds to develop programs in treating those types of cases. Even the brilliant doctors in those hospitals couldn't possibly develop the expertise because they don't see enough cases over time."

How unevenly is experience distributed? Every hospital has radiologists, but only three or four radiologists *in the country* can do the kind of finely detailed scans, called "characterizations," of tiny veins in the brain necessary for a neurosurgeon to effectively remove the small pituitary tumors that cause Cushing's disease. Indeed, according to the Cushing's Tumor Society, only twenty-five endocrinologists in the country truly understand how to treat that complicated disease. Dr. Martin Malawer, an orthopedic surgeon at the Washington Hospital Center in Washington, D.C., specializes in musculoskeletal tumors, or sarcomas, so rare that there are only about two or three thousand of them in a country of 250 million people. Of these, the lion's share are treated by just "a half dozen" doctors, according to Dr. Malawer. Only about seventy centers around the country do liver transplants, but of these, Dr. Nancy Ascher, a leading liver transplant surgeon, would only recommend ten "if my mother needed a new liver." Why? "Because those ten do huge numbers of transplants." A regional hospital might do only a few dozen livers and kidneys in a year — the minimum number required to have an approved transplant program — while Ascher's center, the University of California, San Francisco, Medical Center, will do 110 livers and 220 kidneys in that same year.

Wider experience means greater expertise, which also means sharper diagnoses — as I learned. As Bob and Sheila Miner learned, too, when their thirteen-year-old son suddenly gained twenty-five pounds in a week at tennis camp. The camp nurse maintained that "he was just drinking too much soda." The boy's usual pediatrician scratched his head in bewilderment and told the Miners, "I think I might have seen a case like this ten years ago." Not until the Miners drove to a pediatric nephrologist (kidney expert) at a big teaching hospital in New York City did they find out that their son had a serious kidney problem. The doctor, a Japanese woman, "saw ten cases like that a day," Bob Miner told me, "instead of one in ten years."

"The falsehood that the American public has been sold," says Andrea Hecht, president of the Cushing's Tumor Society, "is that the local community doctor is going to understand and be able to treat anything that comes along. It simply is not true and it's a completely unrealistic expectation of our physicians."

A doctor at a major medical center told me about a young girl who woke up one morning complaining of double vision and weakness. A few hours later, she was "locked in" — awake but completely paralyzed, able to move only her eyes. Locked-in syndrome gets its name from the book *The Count of Monte Cristo,* in which a man is confined in an inflexible suit of armor, with only his eyes showing. Locked-in patients are sometimes thought to be comatose because they can't talk, but their thinking brains are fully functioning and they can communicate with eye movements. ("Look to the left if the answer is 'yes.'")

Doctors quickly determined that the girl's vertebral artery, the main artery to the brain stem, was blocked. It wasn't clear exactly what was causing the blockage, but with no time to waste, they administered an experimental clot-busting drug, TPA. Within a matter of hours, the artery opened up and she began to move. "Actually, I think she's back at school now," says one of her doctors. "She's still weak, but she would have been completely paralyzed, the paralysis would have become permanent, if she hadn't gotten that drug when she did. And at a small community hospital, they wouldn't have figured that out. They wouldn't have the people who know enough about it. I'm using a euphemism here: 'hospital' where I really mean 'doctors.'"

Dr. Louis Caplan, neurologist in chief and a stroke specialist at the New England Medical Center in Boston, told me about another patient, a young schoolteacher, who was brought in from a smaller hospital in deep coma. "She had already had one stroke, and then started to develop dizziness and headache, and then, the next thing anybody knew, she was unconscious." The other hospital didn't have any idea what was happening to her.

Caplan saw signs that something was going wrong in the woman's cerebellum, and subsequent tests showed "a very, very large cerebellar infarct" which had compressed her brain stem. In other words, a massive stroke — the kind of stroke that is fatal in "100 percent" of cases unless it is decompressed immediately. Within two hours, the woman was in the operating room. Without the right set of skills — skills not available at the other hospital — "it might not have been diagnosed that quickly and that accurately," says Caplan, "and if it wasn't diagnosed within twelve hours, she would have been dead."

The medical profession might not take offense at the suggestion that some doctors are better *for certain kinds of ailments* because they have more experience identifying and treating those ailments. That is, after all, the whole rationale behind specialization. A much harder pill for the profession (and, surprisingly, patients) to swallow is that some doctors are better because they are simply more skilled, more knowledgeable, more intelligent — in short, more competent.

No one would argue that all plumbers are equally competent, or all hair dressers, or all teachers. In three years of law school, I learned that all lawyers are certainly not created equal — even all lawyers trained at Harvard Law School. They vary in intelligence, commitment, creativity, and, perhaps most important, intensity — the ability to focus on a problem until it's solved. There is also a particular kind of intelligence — rational, linear — that is best suited to legal work, and those of my classmates who were smart *in that way* simply made better lawyers. They had (there's no other word for it) *aptitude.* Others, whose intelligence tended more toward the intuitive and associative, fared less well. They passed all their courses, of course, some even made high marks, and many went on to join prestigious law firms, but they would never be as good at lawyering as their better-suited classmates.

The same is true of doctors. "It's true in medicine just as it's true in law or professional athletics," says Dr. James Kirklin, director of heart and lung transplantation at the University of Alabama Hospital in Birmingham, who went to Harvard Medical School. "Being bright is one thing, but certain people commit themselves to a higher level of accomplishment while others phase off. I saw an array of people in medical school all of whom, I'm sure, scored well on IQ tests. But how much did they apply themselves, how much did they really want it, how determinedly did they extract all the information and commit themselves to mastering it? Obviously, there was tremendous variation."

Doctors know the truth, but most, unlike Dr. Kirklin, are loath to admit it publicly. Virtually all the prominent physicians I interviewed agreed, as one put it, that "the notion that all doctors are the same isn't just a myth; it is, on its face, a ridiculous notion." Yet they all, like that one, asked not to be quoted on the subject. "It's a very deep-rooted thing in the medical community," says Dr. Peter Scardino, chief of the urology service at the Methodist Hospital in Houston and a prominent urologic oncologist. "Anytime a surgeon gives a talk at a meeting or writes a paper and implies that he can do something that others can't do, or some of us can do something that everybody else can't do, that creates a huge amount of antagonism on the part of the audience. It can almost guarantee that people who would have referred patients to you will, quietly and individually, stop doing it."

Why are doctors afraid of such an obvious truth? Dr. Scardino suggests one possibility. "There is a fear that if one particular doctor is the best in the world for brain tumors, for example, and can do things that nobody else can do, every patient would go to that doctor."

How important are the differences between doctors? The answer depends to some extent on the kind of doctor and the nature of the illness. An internist prescribing drugs for a particular problem is following a formula that is well established and doesn't vary from doctor to doctor or hospital to hospital. Short of outright incompetence, a patient will get the same concentration and dose of medicine regardless of his or her doctor's comparative skill. On the other hand, the success of radiation therapy, which most people think varies little from place to place, is, in fact, incredibly dependent upon the skill of the radiation therapist as well as the quality of the machinery being used.

How important are the differences between doctors? As important as the difference between operable and inoperable. "When I was a resident at M.G.H.," recalls Dr. Scardino, "time after time we saw patients who had been turned down for surgery or were sent to us with a tumor that some doctor had labeled 'inoperable.' We used to say, that doesn't mean the tumor is inoperable, it means *that doctor* can't operate on it."

Nowhere are the differences between doctors more pronounced, or more important, than in surgery. "There are some doctors who can just do operations better than others," says Dr. Kirklin. "It doesn't make any difference whether he's done a hundred or ten, he just does them better." Kirklin is not just talking about pioneering experimental surgeries like interspecies organ transplants, either. Even for a procedure as common as prostate surgery, skills vary widely from surgeon to surgeon.

In prostatectomies (removal of the prostate) for cancer, for example, urologic surgeons try to achieve what they call "negative surgical margins," which is doctorspeak for getting it all out. If a surgeon can achieve negative surgical margins, the chances of the cancer recurring are virtually nil. Positive surgical margins mean the cancer is more likely to return. Currently, almost a third of patients who undergo prostatectomies have positive surgical margins. In addition, prostate surgery can leave a patient incontinent and/or impotent.

"Virtually any urologist in the country can take a prostate gland out," says Dr. Scardino. "Every urologist for generations has gone through training on how to do it. The patient can come into the hospital, have his prostate removed, and go home. Everything's fine. But you need to ask what are the chances that the surgical margins will be positive? That the patient will be incontinent? That the patient will be impotent? So the question for surgeons is not can you take out the prostate, it's can you take out the prostate with a high probability of removing all the cancer and end up with a patient who is not incontinent and not impotent? Now, you've gone from something that every urologist can basically do to something that's extremely difficult."

Ask a typical urologist about the impotence rate of his prostatectomy patients, however, or the incontinence rate, or the positive surgical margin rate, and he probably won't know them; or, if he does, will say he doesn't believe they mean anything. He just knows that he can take out a prostate gland. His patients go home to their lives and are fine. He's sure that his positive surgical margin rate, if he knew it, would be no different than any other doctor's. Same with his impotence rate. And he doesn't believe those surgeons who claim that only two or three percent of their patients are incontinent.

Yet one of the few comparative studies ever undertaken of prostate surgery, by a urologist at the Mayo Clinic, showed that *just*

among the twelve surgeons at Mayo who performed prostatectomies, the rates of incontinence varied radically — from a low of
1 percent to a high of 15 percent. And that was just the range
within one hospital — and a highly reputable one at that. "After
all the courses and all the training and all the experience," says
Dr. Hermes Grillo, "there is just a huge difference from one set of
hands to another set of hands."

With the variation in quality so great, and the consequences so
dire, the search for the right doctor takes on a new and sobering
significance.

FOUR

Looking for Dr. Right

THE TAYLORS NEVER saw that Mayo report. No one did. It was never published. But unlike a lot of patients, the Taylors didn't take anything for granted. The Mayo doctor they flew halfway around the world to see turned out to be "a man of great charm and courtesy and a very compassionate physician," but they were struck by the fact that his name did not appear on any of the most recent articles on the treatment of bone marrow cancer. It wasn't much, but it was enough to make them keep looking. Later, they would learn that he had made his name in the field more than twenty years before and was no longer on the cutting edge of myeloma therapy.

With slides and test results in hand, they continued their "journey of discovery" around the U.S. — Chicago, Boston, Dallas, Phoenix, San Francisco, Seattle — looking at other programs at other hospitals, talking to other doctors, other experts, still not taking anybody's word as the last one. To make sure they missed nothing, they recorded all their interviews on tape. "We asked the doctors if they minded," Melissa Taylor recalls, "and if anyone had said they minded, we wouldn't have stayed." Later, in the solitude of hotel rooms far from home, they reviewed the tapes again and again, writing down unfamiliar words, reading the tea leaves of inflection, struggling to understand what they had heard. Looking for Dr. Right.

Finally, after six weeks of searching, they called Dr. Bart Barlogie. "He took our phone call even before we met him," Harold recalls. "He gave us as long as we wanted on the phone and didn't shy away when we challenged him to explain why his program was better than the others." When they visited him, the Taylors were impressed by the way Barlogie "combined scientific excellence with genuine patient concern"; by his openness, his willingness to inform, his readiness to explain. "We felt we had finally found someone who really focused on this particular problem," recalls Melissa, "and was doing everything he could to move forward the treatment of what had always been an extremely unresponsive disease."

In short, they had found Dr. Right.

And he wasn't at Mayo, or Dana Farber, or M. D. Anderson — all of which the Taylors had visited. He was at the University of Arkansas in Little Rock.

I wasn't as smart as Harold and Melissa Taylor. Maybe it's the difference between entrepreneurs and lawyers: one always looking for new solutions to old problems, the other for old solutions to new problems. Whatever the reason, despite my missteps on the way to Dr. Wohl, despite the buffetings of Morton's neuroma, shoe inserts, and unnecessary crutches, I continued to cling to my Dr. Welby notions about doctors. Partly, I was lulled into complacence by the quality of the doctors I had stumbled onto. Dr. Wohl, a model of self-effacing competence, immediately referred me to Dr. Steven Krane, one of the leading experts on metabolic bone diseases and director of the bone research unit at Massachusetts General Hospital. How could I be in better hands? I didn't need to think about finding the right doctors; they had found me.

Or so I thought.

After a two-week stay in the research wing at M.G.H., I didn't know much more about why my kidneys were leaking phosphorus, but I did find out just how rare my problem was and discovered one of the eternal verities of medicine: "If you *have* to be sick," as Dr. Krane told me in a lighter moment (thinking, I'm sure, that he was cheering me up), "it definitely helps to be sick in an exotic way." In other words, you're much more likely to light your doctor's fire if you're not "just another cardiac infarction." Over the next few months, I was the subject of both grand rounds (a kind of hospital-wide show-and-tell where doctors present their most intriguing/puzzling cases to a room full of colleagues), and a lengthy article in the *New England Journal of Medicine*.

As I pored over the largely unintelligible article for some new nugget of information that might help me better understand what was happening to me, I found it. Amid the whole-body bone scans and single-cell electron micrographs, blood counts and urinalysis results, I found one sentence of chillingly plain English: "If untreated, patient ran the risk of spinal collapse." When I asked Dr. Krane if that meant what I thought it meant, he nodded his head gravely: Best case, paralysis; worst case, death.

Finding out, after the fact, that you've *had* a close brush with death is very different from actually facing it. As with a traveler who misses a plane that later crashes, the elation of escape overwhelms the chill of what-might-have-been. You get the thrill without the dread. I didn't know it at the time, but this was only the first of many close brushes with the Grim Reaper — some of them far closer.

More interesting and less unnerving was the article's discussion of the old question: Why? In a kind of quiz-show conclusion, the authors threw the question of what caused my condition to a panel of doctors. They asked about my dietary habits, my travel history, even my childhood milk consumption. Because adult-onset osteomalacia, like mine, is so extraordinarily rare (only forty reported cases), one of the panelists floated a theory that I had, in fact, been suffering from the disease since childhood but *didn't know it* because the primary symptom, demineralization of the bone, had been kept in check by a prodigious intake of milk. Only after college, when I went to Europe and stopped drinking the white stuff, did the disease finally show itself.

That, at least, was the theory.

As for the *original* cause of the problem, no one even ventured a guess, bizarre or otherwise. So the article ended on a familiar note:

Diagnosis: OSTEOMALACIA

Cause: IDIOPATHIC

How could this be? How could the best minds in medicine not have the answer? I wasn't so much angry at their failure as puzzled. Dr. Paul never said, "I don't know," without sending me on to someone who did. Drs. Casey, Kildare, and Welby never used the word "idiopathic." This was a face of medicine I had never seen before: indecision. Even dire news, I told myself (naively), was better than this limbo of uncertainty; even anger, better than this vacuum of frustration.

But I was still convinced that if *my* doctors didn't know the cause, the cause must not be knowable. So I went on with my life. For more than a year, I took supplements, avoided shaking hands, limited my walking, and wondered if I would ever run again. I would wake up from vivid dreams of sprinting through fields and jumping over fences like a racehorse and think how good it felt, and how familiar, and yet how remote and impossible.

Then, almost two years later, I went to see a doctor about an earache. Detecting some fluid behind the eardrum, the doctor prepared to put a tube through the drum so the fluid could drain — a relatively routine procedure. What he found was anything but routine. The tiny hole he punched in the drum began to jet blood. For the first time in my life, I saw a doctor panic. He didn't run around the room screaming or tearing his hair. It all happened in his eyes. Which only made it scarier.

Within an hour, I was on the table in his operating room being prepped for an emergency procedure. The bleeding was coming from a strange mass of tissue behind the eardrum, and he thought it should come out. Now.

I don't remember asking any questions. It all happened so fast, I scarcely had time to register a reaction. I have a vague memory of a little voice that said, "Eureka," even as they wheeled me into the operating room; a voice that said this, finally, was the answer to the "Why?" that had stumped all the experts; finally, an end to all those "idiopathics." Certainly, there was no time to find another doctor or get a second opinion — or at least I didn't think there was. The doctor said it needed to come out, and the doctor was always right.

So it came out. Along with the hearing in that ear and the feeling on that side of my face. After a few months of numbness, the sensation mostly returned, but the hearing, despite several follow-up reconstructive surgeries, disappeared forever.

All for what? The doctor couldn't guarantee that he had gotten all of it out (whatever it was) — "it was such a bloody mess," he protested. So "it" might come back. And the pathology was inconclusive: The lab couldn't tell what it was or where it came from. The report ended on another familiar note:

Type of Tissue: GRANULAR
Origin: UNKNOWN

Four years later, I was working in Los Angeles writing a PBS series on the Supreme Court and the Constitution with my old law school professor, Archibald Cox, when the numbness returned — only a slight numbness at the corner of my right eye, but a numbness nonetheless. As soon as I recognized it, my heart sank. Convinced that the strange growth in my ear was back, I hurried to the House Clinic, a highly reputable institution in Los Angeles that specializes in ear problems. Like patients since time immemorial, I sat in the waiting room thinking, repeating over and over again the mantra "Such a minor symptom: How serious could it be?"

A CT scan showed how serious.

The growth was back, all right, only bigger and badder than ever. Now, instead of an olive-sized mass, it was an egg. And instead of being wedged in the narrow passage of my ear canal, it was nestled *inside* my skull, up against my brain, like an egg under a chicken. The numbness was caused by pressure on a nerve that ran between the chicken and the egg.

I had a brain tumor.

All the scans and all the reassuring words and all the detailed, demystifying descriptions boiled down to this one irreducible, undigestible, this-can't-be-happening-to-me fact.

I had a brain tumor.

That should have been the start of *my* journey of discovery. If I had been Harold Taylor, it would have been. I would have gone to a medical library and read everything I could find on brain tumors; found out what the doctors meant when they talked about "sarcomas" and "meningiomas" and what the difference was; and where, exactly, was the "right temporal fossa." I would have identified the best specialists in the field and talked to as many of them as I could find, made tapes of the conversations and notes of everything they said that I didn't understand. I would have ferreted out "the centers of excellence" for the treatment of brain tumors, collected my scans and tests, made plane reservations, and embarked on a quest for my Dr. Right.

What *did* I do?

I took the name of the brain surgeon the House Clinic gave me and walked across the street to his office.

In retrospect, it seems like a stunning act of naïveté: to take a referral at face value; to assume that the name on that slip represented someone's conscientious effort to direct me to the best medical care available for my problem — to Dr. Right.

In fact, referrals can be made for any number of reasons — only one of which is what's best for the patient. For example, a hospital struggling to establish a program in, say, angioplasty, will do everything it can to encourage doctors to refer candidates for angioplasty "in-house" — for their program "to practice on," as one doctor put it — even if a better program is available elsewhere. A very prominent surgical oncologist told me that officials at his hospital "get mad" when he tells patients they will be better served by going to a medical oncologist at the nearby university medical center.

Where program-building ends, group loyalty begins. "If a doctor has a reputation as somebody who always refers the difficult, challenging problems outside," says Dr. Peter Scardino, "people start asking, 'Don't you have any confidence in your own medical community?' He's likely to hear about it at the next medical staff meeting. The other specialists in that area are going to say, 'Hey, look, we can do this too, you know.'"

That's exactly what a surgeon told Jeremy Eisen when he was rushed to the hospital with a cerebral hemorrhage. A twenty-one-year-old Dartmouth student, Eisen was spending the weekend at his girlfriend's house in Sharon, Connecticut, when the headache started. "I felt like my brain was in a pneumatic press," he remembers, "like my eyes were going to pop out of my head." By the time he reached the car for the trip to the hospital, his sight was beginning to go. "Everything started getting kind of wavy."

At the little community hospital in Sharon, doctors discovered the hemorrhage and bundled Eisen onto a helicopter headed to the nearest neurological ICU (intensive care unit), in Hartford. The doctors there determined that the hemorrhage had been caused by an AVM (arteriovenous malformation), a weak spot in a blood vessel, and that Eisen would need surgery. "The doctor at Hartford told my parents that they were very capable of doing it there," recalls Eisen. But as more and more doctors made their way to his room, bringing more and more of their students and colleagues, Eisen began to have doubts. "I got the feeling that this was a case that they'd never had before, that it was pretty exciting for them, that it would be like icing on the cake for them to do an AVM operation."

Fortunately, Eisen's mother stepped in to make sure nobody "practiced" on her son. Pam Eisen had spent years caring for a daughter with a rare chromosomal defect, Prader-Willi syndrome, that leaves its victims stunted, mentally retarded, and driven by an appetite so ravenous, so insatiable, that sufferers can literally eat themselves to death. (Once, her daughter saw the picture of a cake on a cake-mix box and ate all the dry mix inside. The family had to put a lock on the kitchen door.) If there was one thing Pam Eisen knew, it was how to research rare medical problems, and how to find the right doctors to treat them. Within days, she had located one of the leading AVM surgeons in the world at Columbia-Presbyterian in New York, and had her son transferred there.

Jeremy Eisen was caught in a "referral loop" — an I-scratch-your-back-you-scratch-mine arrangement in which doctors refer patients back and forth within a closed circle. Loops can be formal or informal; they can be based on institutional priorities or group loyalties or just loose, economic affiliations. One doctor described a typical arrangement this way: "Larry is an oncologist who refers to one or two ENT people, one or two surgeons, one or two heart men, and they all in turn refer their oncology patients back to Larry. Everybody wins."

Everybody except the patient, that is.

Whether the reason is professional rivalry, competitive pressure, economic necessity, or all of the above, the problem with referrals is "part of the fabric of medicine," according to one prominent cancer specialist. "A doctor may send me his mother, but yet he never sends me one of his patients. Think about the ethics of that."

Needless to say, I wasn't thinking about ethics or referral loops or group loyalty or hospital politics or the fabric of medicine as I stumbled out of the House Clinic still reeling from the news. *Brain tumor?!* It's one of those medical phrases that short-circuit the rational mind — like "the plague" in previous centuries or "cancer" in previous decades — an archetype of fatal affliction that elicits universal gasps of horror, revulsion, sympathy, and thank-God-it-wasn't-me relief. What I felt at that moment, however, was more like confusion than horror, a confusion that was one part "this can't be true," one part "it must be true," and one part "what do I do?" The only thing I knew for certain was that I wanted to put a stop to the confusion. So I walked across West Third Street clutching the name they had given me, Dr. Rudolf Heidigger (not his real name, for reasons that will become obvious), in desperate confidence that I was being delivered into the most capable hands available; that if any doctor could rid me of this tumor in my head, he could. After all, a brain surgeon is a brain surgeon is a brain surgeon.

Dr. Heidigger's office occupied the ground floor of a big Victorian house that looked like Mother Bates's place in *Psycho*. The doctor himself was a German man in his fifties, I would say, with an accent like Henry Kissinger's and about as warm. He spent some time looking over my scans, making deep, indecipherable noises as each sheet yielded a new and, I imagined, darker view. Finally, he took a full-scale model of a human skull from the shelf behind his desk and began to explain in his Manhattan-Project accent exactly what he planned to "do for me": He would start by unhinging my jaw ("snap" went the plastic patient), then he would cut out a plate of bone about the size of a demitasse saucer extending from the roof of my mouth up to my ear ("snap" went another piece of plastic). This would give him "comfortable" access to the tumor, he said, which was located roughly two or three inches behind my eye.

I looked at the plastic skull. Half its face was gone.

"I assume you can put all this back together?" I joked lamely.

"Zertainly," said Dr. Heidigger as he fumbled to find the pieces he had removed. "Of course, zere is no vay of telling vat ze neurological damage and scarring vill be."

And that was it. I filled out some forms (especially insurance) and we agreed on a date for the surgery three weeks hence. I walked out of his office convinced that the situation was under control, that I had moved quickly and decisively to bring this new, strange, and terrifying chapter in my life to a quick end.

Fifteen years later, I still can't believe I thought it was that easy; that I could saunter in and out of brain surgery with no more effort than I might bring to a carpet cleaning or cable TV repair. I'm not alone, though. "You wouldn't believe the 'buts' I hear," says Andrea Hecht, who, as president of the Cushing's Tumor Society, hears from a lot of people who have just been told, as I was, that they are facing major brain surgery. "'*But* I don't know where to look,' '*but* it's too expensive,' '*but* it's too much trouble,' '*but* what about the inconvenience.' Imagine! This is their life they're talking about!"

Hecht tells the story of a woman from Tennessee who called to say she was scheduled for pituitary surgery by a neurologist. She had never had an MRI scan done; there wasn't even a clear diagnosis, but her surgery was only two days away. By her own telling, Hecht "went crazy." "I said, you absolutely have got to call this surgery off," she says, "there are *neurosurgeons* who don't know how to do this procedure. But a neurologist!" The woman did cancel the surgery, and Hecht put her in touch with a qualified surgeon at Vanderbilt, but she worries about all the other patients out there who don't pick up the phone, and all the other 'buts.'

Why do so many people, like me, walk blindly into one of the most important decisions of their lives? Why will the same people who throw weeks of effort into finding the right mechanic for their car or the right hairdresser or the right housepainter take whatever doctor they're referred to without asking a single question? Is it simplemindedness, as some doctors suggested to me: a desire to get it over with, "get it out" — as quickly, painlessly, and thoughtlessly as possible? Is it another expression of the "doctor knows best" syndrome: Patients need to have trust, need to believe that the doctor can make them better, and to look elsewhere undermines that trust? Or is it, as one patient suggested, the fear that a more aggressive doctor might demand more difficult sacrifices, like giving up alcohol, or present the patient with more difficult choices? "A lot of patients don't want to hear that their case isn't simple," says one doctor, "and above all, they don't want to make choices. They want the doctor to make the choices for them."

David Peretz, a psychiatrist on the faculty of Columbia University who specializes in treating terminally ill patients and their families, suggests that some patients don't think they're worth the trouble and effort involved in seeking out better medical care. "Some people, when they get bad news, give up right there," says Peretz. "It may not show on the surface, but they regress to a dependent position. They want somebody else — anybody will suffice — to tell them what to do. Then there is the masochistic personality — people who are ready to accept that the ax they've been expecting has finally fallen. And those are the ones who will resist doing very much about their situation."

Whatever its cause, this strange aversion to pursuing the best medical care, no matter how grave the consequences, strikes people at all economic and social levels. "I am appalled," says Dr. Nicholas Kouchoukos, chief cardiothoracic surgeon at the Jewish Hospital at Washington University Medical Center in St. Louis, "by professional people, highly educated people, successful people, who don't know even where to start looking for the solution to a complicated medical problem, or sometimes a not-so-complicated problem." Dr. Louis Caplan, the chief neurologist at the New England Medical Center, suggests that maybe the "helplessness" that comes over otherwise self-possessed, successful people at times of life-threatening illness is related to their privileged status.

"Privileged people assume that life will be easy and that things will happen as they want them to happen, and therefore, once some catastrophe hits, they just can't cope with it."

One way to understand why people don't search out the best medical care more aggressively is to look more closely at the excuse that's most commonly used to avoid that search — the biggest 'but,' so to speak: "I don't want to travel." In my own case, even though I was on the opposite coast from my real home, I can remember the warm wave of reassurance I felt when the doctor at the House Clinic told me Dr. Heidigger's office was directly across the street. It wasn't much, but at the time, trying to cope with terrible news in a strange city, "home" was wherever anybody offered help.

Dr. Thomas Petty, a leading emphysema specialist at Presbyterian – St. Luke's in Denver, calls this the "homing instinct" — the tendency of people who are sick to want to be home, or close to home, or at least near family. The more serious the illness, the stronger the homing instinct. Unfortunately, the homing instinct often interferes with the search for the best medical care. Almost without exception, the best care for most serious illnesses is at institutions that have track records of taking care of large volumes of patients with those illnesses. Just one example: The Whipple procedure is an operation performed by gastrointestinal surgeons. At small, local hospitals, the mortality rate for Whipple procedures is 25 percent. At large medical centers, the rate is 5 percent. Studies of stroke victims have shown again and again that the chance of having not just a survivorship, but a good quality survivorship, is considerably better at large medical centers with experience in treating stroke victims.

There are, of course, some things that local hospitals do perfectly well, even superlatively. "If a patient just has simple pneumonia," says Dr. James Kirklin, the heart transplanter at the University of Alabama, "and is coughing up some stuff, any hospital can take care of that. But if they have devastating lung injury, both lungs out on a mechanical ventilator, they shouldn't be in a small community hospital." Dr. Donald Skinner, a urologic oncologist at the Los Angeles County/University of Southern California Medical Center, gave me the well-documented example of a rare malignancy that attacks children, called Wilms' tumor. Studies have shown that a child with Wilms' tumor has a much better chance of survival if he or she is treated in a children's medical center than if left in a community hospital. "And I think you would find that true with most serious conditions," adds Dr. Skinner.

Despite all this, despite all the evidence and the studies and the urgings even of the medical community, people still cling to home. No matter how serious the illness, no matter how much better the care or the survival rates elsewhere, the "homing" instinct wins out. I have a friend, a lawyer in a small West Coast town, who was diagnosed with prostate cancer. He immediately scheduled surgery with a local GP who wasn't even board certified in general surgery. Why? "So my family can come visit me in the hospital," he said. Several of his friends, including me, urged him to see one of the experts at Los Angeles County or U.C.L.A. or Stanford or the University of California at San Francisco — all within driving distance. We even gave him the names of the best urologic oncologists at those centers. I pleaded my own sad history: how I had learned the lesson the hard way; how much better he would feel knowing he was in expert hands; at least he could rest assured that, whatever happened, he had given himself the best chance of success, done everything he could.

He went ahead and had the surgery done locally. The outcome was, in the euphemistic jargon of medicine, "unfavorable." After a year of bed-bound suffering, he died, leaving a wife and two small children. Perhaps the result would have been the same at Stanford or Los Angeles County or wherever, but his family will always be haunted by the fact that he could have done more to save himself.

Some people argue that the issue is money: The cost of seeing distant doctors at major medical centers, even just for consultation, is prohibitive, and may not be covered by insurance. But money isn't really the issue. Denial comes in every tax bracket. I talked to a man who was looking for a radiation oncologist. "My wife just had surgery for a brain tumor at the local medical center in Southern California where we live," he said. "The tumor turned out to be malignant and we need somebody to do the radiation." I asked him if he could possibly get to San Francisco, where I knew there were several world-class radiation oncologists. At that point, his sister, who was also on the phone, jumped in. "Well, I should let you know that my brother's a very senior executive with the Sony Corporation," she said, "and he has access to a private jet." And I was thinking, You're a senior executive with the Sony Corporation, with a private jet, and you took your wife to the closest hospital for *brain surgery?*

"People will go to Europe because it's a good year for wine," says Dr. Scardino, "but they won't leave town for a doctor. It's astounding." Dr. Scardino tells a story from his hometown, Savannah, Georgia, where his father was also a doctor. "There was a very wealthy man — one of my brothers used to date his daughter — who had a heart attack on the tennis court and was taken to the local hospital. They couldn't figure out what to do and they fooled around with him for about ten days in the coronary care unit and he died. It was unbelievable. In a minute his family could have called for a medevac helicopter or a private plane to fly him to Houston and had Michael DeBakey [the celebrated heart surgeon] personally operate on him, yet he was perfectly happy to die there in the local coronary care unit. And his family had no problem with it. It never occured to them that anything different could be done."

When asked to explain such bizarre behavior, one doctor I spoke to suggested that perhaps people are intimidated by big institutions. "They know research is done at these places and they're afraid they're going to be experimented on; they'll be treated like experimental animals. At a local hospital, they think they're more likely to be treated like a human being, not just a number on a clipboard." Dr. Scardino himself suggests that maybe trust is the issue; that when people face a serious illness, they turn naturally to the people and the community they know and the doctors who have taken care of them in the past. "People feel that if they're very ill and they do die, they want their family to be there," says Scardino. "They don't want to be in some remote place and die in a hospital where nobody knows who they are, with most of their family miles and miles away. They're afraid to die alone."

So, finally, it isn't about money. It isn't about convenience or confidence or even trust. Finally, it's about fear. Fear and denial. Dr. Bennett Stein, one of the premier neurosurgeons in the world, has seen it in every guise. "It comes out in different ways," he says. "The local hospital is more convenient, they don't like the offices, they don't want to hear that there could be bad news, they don't want to hear that the operation might be twelve hours instead of three. It all adds up to one thing: 'It's not that bad.'"

In my own case, I have no doubt that denial is what allowed me to breeze in and out of Dr. Heidigger's office with no more concern and little more time than a visit to the dentist. I was whistling through the graveyard of my fear, coping with an enormous event by denying its enormity; pretending it was really just a simple task. Anything that can be taken care of in a few easy steps — find a doctor, get an operation — can't be as momentous as your fear wants to make it.

And no one is immune from fear; nothing can inoculate you from denial — not wealth, not success, not even experience. "When faced with a potentially catastrophic medical problem," says Dr. Robert Brumback, an orthopedic surgeon specializing in trauma at the University of Maryland in Baltimore, "even people who have already experienced the importance of getting to the right doctor for something really important just sort of lose control. They want to deal with it without thinking, so they'll stay with whatever doctor whose office they happen to have landed in." As an example, Dr. Brumback cites the case of a seventy-six-year-old woman — "healthy as a horse and bright as a tack" — who was diagnosed with Barlow's syndrome, a floppy heart valve that left her short of breath. Even though the woman's son was a prominent orthopedic surgeon, she never consulted him or anybody else as she scheduled heart surgery. Finally, two days before the operation, she called her son — Dr. Robert Brumback.

"Two days before the valve replacement," recalls Brumback, who lives in Baltimore, only a half hour away from his mother, "she phones me and says she's going to have open-heart surgery. It was another form of denial. She didn't want me to get involved. That would have made it seem like a bigger deal. People often say they're minimizing the seriousness of something because they want to spare others the agony, but I think often it's their own agony they're trying to spare."

Even behind the simple, seemingly straightforward reluctance to travel in search of better medical care lurks the spectre of denial. Dr. Andrew von Eschenbach, one of the country's leading urologic surgeons at one of the country's leading cancer treatment centers, M. D. Anderson in Houston, believes that when people refuse to seek treatment for a life-threatening illness at a major medical center, they often talk about distance and family and home, but they're really saying something very different. "I walk out of church on Sunday and somebody tells me about a person that has recently been diagnosed as having cancer and they're being treated over at a small community hospital," says von Eschenbach. "And you ask yourself, how in God's name could they be sitting here in the shadow of M. D. Anderson and seek treatment for cancer at some rinky-dink community hospital? It just doesn't compute. And then you realize what they're really saying is '*My cancer's not that bad*. People only go to places like M. D. Anderson if they're at death's door. But my cancer is nowhere near that bad and we can just take care of it with a little penicillin here at my neighborhood hospital. I'll only go to a place like that when my cancer is *really* bad and everything else has failed. I can do that then, but I don't need to do it now.'"

I spoke to a thirty-eight-year-old woman who was told by her family physician that she had lung cancer. She described him as a "wonderful man, about to retire" who had been her family doctor for as long as she could remember. He gave her the name of a surgeon in the same hospital and, like me, she "just went along with whatever he said." She didn't even see the surgeon until the day of her operation. Later, after she began radiation treatments, she found herself driving by Memorial Sloan-Kettering in New York City, another of the premier cancer centers in the world, and she thought, "God, I sure hope I don't end up there."

Like me, she had to learn the hard way. Within a year, she was admitted to Sloan-Kettering.

Dr. Heidigger never did perform his "face-lift" brain surgery on me. When I called home to report on our meeting, my parents insisted on flying to Los Angeles, both to be with me for the surgery and to make their own assessment of the doctor who would soon be massaging their son's brain. After Heidigger repeated his show-and-tell with the plastic skull for them, my father, a skeptical businessman like Harold Taylor, turned to me and said in horror and disbelief, "He wants to take your face off." That was the first time it really registered with me: Yes, indeed, that was exactly what he wanted to do.

At my father's urging — "There must be another way," he insisted — I went to see a big-name neurosurgeon at U.C.L.A., a major medical center with a national reputation (which, while not across the street, was only a few miles away). But that was as far as I went. I hadn't learned my lesson yet. Without any more searching or studying or questioning (after all, my father was satisfied), I scheduled surgery at U.C.L.A.

Lying in the hospital bed the night before the operation, I

tried, unsuccessfully, to stay calm — sleep being a lost cause. It's only brain surgery, I told myself. I had already been through one operation for this tumor, how much worse could it be? Then, about two o'clock — a very lonely time in a hospital — when I was too tired to keep them under control any longer, the questions started coming: Did I do everything I should have? Was there somebody else I should have seen or talked to? Was this the right operation? Was the right doctor doing it? And on and on.

Two o'clock in the morning, only hours before the white coats come to take you away, is a very bad time to start having second thoughts. At dawn, I was still wide awake, questions still hurtling through my head, when they wheeled me off to the operating room.

And what an operation it was. It may not have been the mutilating extravaganza that Dr. Heidigger proposed, but it wasn't ear surgery either. Instead of removing my face, the doctor cut a plate out of my skull like the lid on a jack-o'-lantern, then fished around for the elusive growth. I remember nothing about the operation, of course, and little about the recovery except my father's tie (he was wearing one I had given him, and I recognized it when I first opened my eyes after surgery — which, in his anxiety, he took as a sign that the operation had been a complete success); and an overpowering thirst, which the ICU nurse would satisfy only with occasional chips of ice doled out like sips from the Grail.

At first, the results of all this agony — and the long recovery to follow — looked encouraging. Not only did the symptoms, the numbness, go away, but the culprit was finally identified. Blessed with a large sample of the "granular" stuff scooped from my skull, the U.C.L.A. pathology lab identified it as a hemangiopericytoma — a word which I quickly learned to pronounce to impress my doctors and later to spell to impress my insurance company. The good news about this mouthful, according to my doctor, was that it was generally "benign." (This was before I learned how misleading a term "benign" can be. No tumors are truly "benign" in the nonmedical sense of the word. Some are just slower-growing than others —*less* malignant, not *un*-malignant. In the end, a cancer is a cancer.)

Identifying the tumor had another benefit. It positively established the link that I had always suspected between the growth in my head and the osteomalacia in my bones. Hemangiopericytomas belong to a family of tumors (neuroendocrine tumors, they're called) known to secrete hormone-like substances that throw the body's chemistry out of whack. For years, this tumor had been pumping something into the bloodstream that "tricked" my kidneys with false chemical messages, causing them to dump phosphorus out through my urine even though my bones were hungry for it.

So the cracks in my feet had in fact been caused by a tumor in my head.

There was bad news, too, though. First, the operation had left me with a number of "deficits" (more euphemistic medicalese), some of which would go away, like a shaved head with a huge, crescent-shaped scar and local numbness where the skull plate had been removed; and some of which would not, like loss of control of the muscles on the right side of my face, resulting in an asymmetrical bite, a lopsided smile, and a puckerless kiss.

But the worse news was that I couldn't be sure it was over.

What hemangiopericytomas lack in malignancy, they make up for in tenacity. Because they are very vascular tumors, meaning that they consist mostly of clouds of tiny blood vessels, they tend to be diffuse, hard to isolate, messy to extract, pointless to radiate, and almost impossible to eradicate. "Think of it as the tortoise of tumors," said my doctor, trying to be upbeat (although I knew well who had won the race between the tortoise and the hare).

In other words, no matter how confident he was that he had gotten it all — and he was confident — he couldn't be sure.

More than anything, I had hoped that the operation would

bring an end to the uncertainty. The promise of it, even the possibility of it, had made all the risks acceptable. Instead, I was left
with a skewed smile, a crescent scar, a lame bite, and a life still in
limbo.

Would the outcome have been different if I had done what
Harold Taylor did? Would my story have ended here if I had
seized control of my medical fate more aggressively and made the
kind of exhaustive search for Dr. Right that the Taylors made?
It's impossible to tell, of course. I do know that after a year-long
course of high-dose chemotherapy at the University of Arkansas
(for which the Taylors rented an apartment in Little Rock and set
up housekeeping half a world away from home), Harold Taylor
has "no active disease." Without a trace of protein in his urine —
the telltale sign of bone marrow cancer — he appears to have
beaten the odds and survived a disease that is, in all but a few
cases, a death sentence.

I also know that Harold Taylor, whatever happens, will never
have to ask "what if?" "I think it is dishonest of anybody to say
that they have completely conquered a cancer like this," he says,
"and I won't pretend that I don't have moments of apprehension
about it coming back. But knowing that I've done everything I
can, knowing that I've done the best I can, knowing that I've
given myself the best chance I can, that makes it possible for me to
sleep easy at night."

I, on the other hand, had just begun my journey; endured only
the first of many sleepless nights.

FIVE

The Last Word

WHEN I TELL the story of Harold Taylor and his transoceanic search for Dr. Right, people often argue that it was easy for him. He was rich and well connected. He could afford to fly around from hospital to hospital, interviewing doctors (at, what, $200 a crack); leave his business and move to Arkansas for six months. Like so many things in life, they say, the dogged pursuit of the best medical care is a luxury only the rich can afford.

My response is always the same: That's denial talking. And to prove it, I tell them another story: the story of Louise Enoch.

Louise was a twenty-four-year-old single mother raising her only daughter, Tamara, on nothing more than love and the modest but steady pay she earned at a Safeway grocery store in northern Virginia. It was April 1982, and Tamara was in third grade, with long blond hair and the irrepressible energy of an eight-year old. She had entered a rope-jumping marathon to raise money for the local heart association; the longer she jumped, the more money she raised. She jumped for three hours — longer than any of her classmates — but still Louise was surprised when she came home limping.

"The gym teacher thinks I have a pulled muscle," Tamara said. Louise was skeptical, but hoped a hot bath and a good night's sleep would help. They didn't. The next morning, Tamara was still limping and Louise noticed that when she put her feet up "one knee was higher than the other." Fearing that she might have fractured a bone, Louise rushed her daughter to the emergency room at Prince William Hospital, a small public community hospital, where they took an x-ray. Mother and daughter were just about to leave when the radiologist asked to speak to Louise alone. "There may be a growth on the bone in your daughter's leg," he told her. "I think you should take her to an orthopedist."

"Okay," said Louise. "I'll make an appointment."

"I don't think you understand, Mrs. Enoch," said the radiologist gravely. "You need to go now."

So instead of going home, mother and daughter walked across the street to the office of an orthopedic surgeon. After looking at the scans, he, too, asked to speak to Louise alone. "Your daughter has a malignant tumor," he told her. "We need to put her in the hospital immediately." With startling speed, faster than she could process the unfolding events, Louise arranged for her parents to bring some clothes to the hospital and Tamara settled into her room. "She thought it was neat," Louise remembers. "This was her first time ever in a hospital and she was playing with the remote control on the TV and the motor on the bed and she thought it was a lot of fun." Not until the nurse came to give Tamara her first shot did the gravity of it all begin to sink in. Both mother and daughter cried.

But that was nothing compared to what happened the next day. After more tests and scans, the doctors took Louise out into the hall and told her that they had confirmed it: Tamara had a malignant tumor in her leg. What did that mean? Louise wanted to know. The leg would have to be amputated, they said. And even then, the cancer would eventually kill her. How long would it take? She would probably be dead within two years, they said.

When Louise started to protest, they cautioned her: "You need to be realistic about this, Mrs. Enoch."

Louise turned away from them and faced the wall. Just in time. The explosion of tears knocked her to her knees. Then she collapsed completely. When she came to, she was sitting in a chair in a different room with her own mother standing over her.

Eventually, Louise worked up the courage to face her daughter. When she saw that bright, trusting face, she almost lost control again. But she found the strength to say the word: "cancer." Tamara didn't have to be reminded that her great-grandmother had just died of that same, strange word. "Does that mean I'm going to die, too?" she asked.

Louise swallowed the great ball of tears that rose inside her. "I don't know, honey," she finally said. "It's really in God's hands. But I'm going to do everything within my power to make sure you don't."

Louise Enoch set out immediately to make good on that promise. She started by finding a bone cancer specialist at the Children's National Medical Center in Washington to review Tamara's case. From the beginning, she had been uncomfortable with the orthopedic surgeon the hospital referred her to — "I felt he wasn't compassionate," she recalls — and the new specialist confirmed her suspicions. Where the orthopedist had seen a second tumor on Tamara's spine, the Washington specialist saw nothing. "After that," she says, "I wasn't going to allow that man to do any kind of cutting on my daughter."

To find a new surgeon, Louise went to the library and searched through every magazine article and book she could find on bone cancer. Every time she saw a doctor's name, she would scribble it down in her spidery cookbook handwriting, then go home and call. It was through that process (and with the help of the cancer specialist at Children's) that she found Dr. Martin Malawer, the orthopedic tumor surgeon at the Washington Hospital Center with a unique specialty: saving limbs. "Most of my cases are patients who would have had amputations," says Dr. Malawer, whose procedure combines massive orthopedic, plastic, and vascular surgery, elaborate prostheses, and chemotherapy. "At first, most people thought I was crazy. They would say, 'Why don't you just amputate? Why do you do all this?' Now it's the standard of care for these tumors."

On an Easter weekend, Louise and Malawer met. "He said he did a pioneering type of surgery," she remembers, "and Tamara would be the youngest patient he had ever attempted it on, but he thought that he could save her leg and her life. This was the first time anyone had said anything like that, and it was like a ray of sunlight after days of rain."

What Louise Enoch knew by intuition and motherlove (nature and nurture, so to speak), I had to struggle for years to learn. Even after my close call with Dr. Heidigger in Los Angeles, I continued to believe that the doctors knew best and that my only duty as a patient was to make myself available to them. Unsure of the possibility of a recurrence, and determined not to let the tumor catch me by surprise again, I began making yearly pilgrimages to the frozen Lourdes of American medicine, the Mayo Clinic in Rochester, Minnesota. Mayo is one of those quasi-mythical places to baby boomers like me; as potent, evocative, and distant a destination as Hollywood or Disneyland or Cape Canaveral in the geography of a midwestern upbringing. It was the place where kings and potentates, movie stars and moguls, went when they got sick — really sick — sick with diseases that no one talked about to gradeschoolers in the 1950s. Until my parents started going there for annual checkups in the 1970s, I had never personally known any Mayo patients, only read about them in newspapers and magazines. I didn't even know that Mayo took "normal" patients.

My father is the one who urged me to go and, on my first visit, showed me around the labyrinth of underground passages that connect the clinic's many buildings, and initiated me in "the Mayo way." Whether it's the discipline imposed by Minnesota's grueling winters or the founders' roots in Presbyterian rectitude, I don't know, but Mayo tends to treat its patients the old-fashioned way: like children. Specifically, children on a short leash. Combine that junior-high-school paternalism with a Scandinavian fetish for order and waiting-room delays that make one nostalgic for the streamlined Soviet bureaucracy, and you have the Mayo way.

By the time of my first visit, in 1982, one year after the surgery at U.C.L.A., most of the postoperative problems had faded. I had a few new bumps and hollows on my head where the skull bone had healed in unexpected ways, I had little feeling on the right side of my face or tongue, and every time my eye closed, my chin twitched (something the doctors called "anomalous re-inner-vation"). Months of therapy for my jaw muscles had finally made it possible for me to get my mouth around a Big Mac, but had done little to correct a facial asymmetry that made me feel like the Elephant Man even as my friends stoutly insisted it was hardly noticeable.

Every year, I would brave the arctic cold and report to Rochester for a battery of scans and tests that lasted three or four days; and every year they would give me the same clean bill of health: no sign of a recurrence. Every year, from 1982 to 1986, the scans were clear.

There was just one problem. The strange blood condition — low phosphorus, high calcium — and the bone condition it caused, osteomalacia, were still present. Everyone seemed to agree that the tumor had caused these other problems, but no one could explain why, if the tumor was gone, the problems persisted. Whenever I pressed the question, the doctors at Mayo would throw up their hands and order another round of tests. (Was there generalized kidney damage? Were my parathyroid glands working?) I would have pursued the mystery further (and, in retrospect, should have) but I was feeling better than I had in years.

The vitamin D and phosphorus supplements, while not a cure, were keeping my bones from cracking, so I could ride my bike in Central Park, walk for miles, even play squash, all without pain for the first time since college, and confident that I was doing everything I could to keep it that way.

No wonder the events of December 1986 came as such a bolt out of the blue. In a single night, the night of our editor's Christmas party, I went from feeling the best (and safest) I had in years, to a drooling, babbling basket case who couldn't even smile right.

No wonder the first place I wanted to go was back to the Mayo Clinic, where I had been given all those clean bills of health. But I had learned my lesson in California. Or so I thought. When I returned from Rochester with the grim news that the tumor was inoperable, I remembered Dr. Heidigger and the last round of grim news. This time, I didn't need a push from my father. I immediately set out to get another opinion. Maybe, just maybe, all those tundra pundits were wrong. Wrong about the tumor being suddenly malignant, wrong about its rapid growth, but most of all wrong about those three months.

Whether out of despair, desperation, or just sheer distance, I didn't give a thought to any of the usual excuses patients offer for not seeking second opinions. I didn't care about offending my current doctors. ("When people come to me for a second opinion," says Dr. Michael Sorrell, the gastroenterologist at the University of Nebraska, "they often ask me not to talk to their doctors about their problem because they don't want to hurt the primary caregivers' feelings.") I recognized and accepted the seriousness of my problem. ("The act of getting another opinion," says Dr. Madelon Baranoski, the former army nurse, "is accepting that your illness is more serious than you want to believe it is.") And I was willing to put up with the inevitable hassles. ("To get a second opinion," says a prominent patient advocate, "you may have to fight to get your records, fight for cooperation from the office staff. And you have to do it at a time when you can barely keep things together. For patients facing a difficult illness, even mortality, it's sometimes more than they can bear.")

Whatever the usual excuses (I don't want to think about it; I don't want to make choices; and, of course, it's not that bad), I was determined not to repeat the mistake I had made in California; determined to see if, in some way, Mayo had failed me. After all, this was exactly the kind of "surprise attack" that I had expected my annual treks north to prevent.

And that's when I made my next mistake.

Where does one go to get a second opinion after Mayo? What's left after you've seen the best? The only institution in the New York area with a reputation equal to the Mayo Clinic's was Memorial Sloan-Kettering, a hospital/cancer reseach center on Manhattan's Upper East Side affiliated with New York Hospital and Cornell Medical School. I started with a lowly neurologist, who listened sympathetically as I struggled to tell my story, looked at my Mayo scans, ordered some more scans, then bounced me "upstairs" to a young neurosurgeon, who listened to my story again, then bounced me farther upstairs to a world-renowned neurosurgeon and one of Sloan-Kettering's pooh-bahs. The question that followed me up this ladder of seniority was simple: Was my tumor operable? The answer from the top: No. The doctors at Mayo had been right on that score.

Those same doctors had also told me that radiation was my only option—although they held out little hope for its success. Were they right about that, too? I went to see the chief of neuro-radiation at Sloan-Kettering, Dr. Louis Harrison. The waiting room outside his office was filled mostly with bald young kids of glum countenance and indistinguishable gender, all waiting to be radiated. Most kept their hats and caps and heavy coats on (it was winter outside, too) to hide their pale bareness. A few wore sunglasses over hollow eyes. They didn't talk and barely moved. In the last bleak week of December, in the trough between holidays, in a big gray city, people in waiting rooms everywhere look bedraggled: Penn Station, City Hall, any subway platform. But this group was a different kind of bedraggled altogether. For the first time since my mouth stopped working, I felt lucky.

Dr. Harrison was an exceptionally patient and thoughtful guide through the thicket of questions about the promises and dangers of radiation therapy. He confirmed that the kind of tumor I had, hemangiopericytoma, was exceedingly rare. So rare, in fact, that there really wasn't much clinical data available on how it would respond to radiation treatment. In fact, off the top of his head, he couldn't think of *any* such data. In other words, radiation might be the only solution, but there was no hard evidence that it was a solution at all.

Indeed, there was some indication that it wasn't. Because radiation therapy works by disrupting the reproductive process of the cells that it bombards, it tends to work best on cells that reproduce rapidly — like malignant cancer cells. Or hair cells. The faster growing the tumor, the more effective the radiation. But hemangiopericytomas are typically very slow-growing tumors (remember the tortoise and the hare). On the other hand, the doctors at Mayo had concluded that my tumor was now malignant — or at least less benign. Suddenly and inexplicably (idiopathic, again), my odd, sluggish reptile of a tumor had been transformed into the fierce, racing rodent of cancer. How else to explain its sudden appearance after years of clear scans and clean bills of health? If the tumor had turned malignant, then radiation might just work. But if Mayo was wrong, if the tumor was still slow-growing, then the radiation might trigger more aggressive growth — turn a benign tumor malignant. Finally, radiation generally works better on small tumors than big tumors. Mine was big.

What was the bottom line?

In the absence of clinical trials, said Dr. Harrison, logic indicated that radiation therapy "did not have a high probability of success" against my tumor.

So Mayo was right again.

But that was just a deduction, Harrison emphasized, not a prediction. "I wish I could tell you yea or nay," he said, with the candor that I have come to appreciate most in doctors. "I wish I could assure you that it will do this good or that harm. But I can't. There simply is not the data out there. This tumor is too rare." When a doctor doubts whether the procedure *that he specializes in* will help — when a surgeon doesn't vigorously recommend surgery — that's the time to listen.

Benign, malignant; fast-growing, slow-growing; big, small. Suddenly my life depended on solving a problem in advanced calculus with four unknown variables. And I didn't even know calculus. How could I make an informed decision when, even after seeing a dozen doctors, I didn't really know what I was facing? There was one thing, however, that all my doctors agreed on: To get a better idea of how my tumor would respond to radiation, I had to see Jerome Posner. He was the one person, the *only* person, who could tell me what I needed to know — the one person who knew more about tumors like mine than anyone else on the planet. Posner was the ultimate authority, a man whose reputation in the world of tumors was nonpareil; a legend among doctors, both for the breadth of his knowledge and the depth of his insight. At the East Coast Olympus of cancer treatment, Posner was the tumor Zeus.

When I told Phil Donahue about the impending audience with Dr. Posner, he asked to come along. Partly, he wanted to show his support for me in what was obviously a trying time, and partly he just wanted to meet this "tumor guru," as he called him.

I told him I appreciated the offer, but I didn't think it was such a good idea.

Today, I would never walk into a doctor's office alone. The more important the subject, the more essential I think it is to have another pair of ears in attendance. At the time, however, it would never have occurred to me. I had been seeing doctors alone since I kicked my mother out of Dr. Paul's office for my pre–ninth grade football physical. Twenty years later, on that fateful Christmas trip to Mayo, my mother had offered to accompany me; but, as usual, I turned her away. "Oh, no, you don't need to come," I said, trying not to alarm her. Steve had also offered to fly to Rochester. "But then my mother would feel left out," I told him. (Later, back in New York, he did accompany me to Dr. Harrison's office, but I made him stay outside in that waiting room filled with sad, silent children.)

Why was I so reluctant to accept the kindness of company? What was I hiding? Or hiding from? At the time, I would have said it was just a need for privacy (what could be more private than cancer?). Or, as I told my mother, I just didn't want to burden anyone. But, looking back, I think the real problem was vulnerability. Vulnerability and control. I didn't want to be seen at my most vulnerable and I wanted to control who knew what about my "problem." I could control it in order to protect others (like my parents, who didn't "need" to know about the three months); or to protect myself ("Poor Greg, he only has three months"). If others had been with me at Mayo that day, I would have had to worry about their reactions (panic? depression? surrender? denial?) as well as my own, their needs as well as my own; the courtesies as well as the calamity.

In fact, I was making things worse — for me and for those around me. I was depriving myself of their help, and them of the knowledge they needed to help me. At the simplest level, it's a matter of "two heads are better than one." Harold and Melissa Taylor, unlike me, understood that from the start. "I was there to help Harold analyze what was being said," recalls Melissa, who joined her husband in doctors' offices across America, "because the emotion of it keeps you from hearing things you don't want to hear, and that could be important. No matter how brilliant you may be, you're under an enormous amount of pressure and anxiety, and this is highly complicated stuff, just the vocabulary alone. And you don't have the luxury of sitting around for six months to figure it all out."

There is a deeper kind of help, of course, that meets a deeper kind of need. "People perform their bravest if they feel someone appreciates their bravery," says Melissa, "and, of course, it helps if someone is nudging them along the way. I was determined to do both those things for Harold."

I, on the other hand, was prepared to forgo help of any kind in the pursuit of privacy, and in a desperate, belated, and ultimately misguided effort to reassert some semblance of control over my disintegrating life.

Luckily, Phil wouldn't take no for an answer.

Arriving at Memorial Sloan-Kettering in a limousine accompanied by a celebrity only heightened the sense of pilgrimage. Like Mohammed to the mountain, I had come to receive the last word on my tumor, the ultimate second opinion, from the tumor guru himself. As Phil and I walked through the halls, heads turned, conversations stopped, gurneys braked. Patients in wheelchairs who hadn't even looked up in months came to life and paddled after us. On the crowded elevator, no one said a word, but everyone was smiling. I asked Phil to stop off at Dr. Harrison's waiting room on the way to the mountaintop. I wanted him to see the children there; and them to see him. The effect, both ways, was what I expected. The hollow-eyed children crowded around him, so grateful for a moment of glitter in their gray lives; and Phil, whose powers of empathy are epic and real, gave them every kindness, then turned and left before they saw his tears.

The secretaries in Dr. Posner's office could barely contain themselves. All business stopped as Phil worked the little crowd of patients and workers like the professional he was, flattering, sympathizing, commiserating, joking. Someone produced the inevitable autograph book, which Phil signed with a felt-tipped flourish and an embarrassed smile.

Guru Posner was a different story. As soon as his starry-eyed secretary ushered us into his office, I could sense the tension in the antiseptic hospital air. He was a bald, gnomish man with a stiff, standoffish manner, the kind of person you might expect to find manning a remote lighthouse or watching over an archive of rare and rarely used manuscripts. In a way, he was both to me. I could tell that he was bothered by Phil's presence. Having never brought a second into a doctor's office, I immediately felt called upon to defend him. "He's a close and concerned friend," I said, "who just happens to have a recognizable face."

It didn't help. Perhaps Posner was worried about violating doctor-patient confidentiality, I thought. "Anything you can say to me," I assured him, "you can say in front of Mr. Donahue."

That didn't help, either. For the rest of the meeting, Posner looked at Phil only rarely and always with a suspicious squint. Did he think we were doing an exposé on doctors? Was he looking for a hidden camera?

As the meeting wore on, I realized that part of the problem was sheer vanity. (Yes, doctors have egos. They couldn't do what they do without them.) As perhaps the number one oncologist in America, Posner was accustomed to being the last word, the opinion of last resort, and he played the part of celebrated guru with obvious relish. These were not just pearls dropping from his lips, these were diamonds. He was accustomed to being the only celebrity in the room, or certainly in his own office. And he didn't like sharing his spotlight with a talk-show host, no matter how many times his secretary called and asked if anybody wanted coffee.

And just what were these pearls, er, diamonds, of wisdom that we had come to the mountaintop to hear? The tumor was, indeed, malignant. It was also, indeed, inoperable. Radiation was, indeed, the only possible solution, but no, indeed, it wasn't very likely to succeed.

In other words, Mayo was right.

The air of celebrity and finality that had shone on our arrival cast a pall over our departure. As high as I had been coming in, higher and more optimistic than in weeks, that's how low I was going out, more hopeless and despondent than ever. Phil did his best to cheer me up. He even invited me to a dinner party at his Fifth Avenue apartment after the New Year's holiday. But nothing helped.

I spent a despondent New Year's Eve, alternately working feverishly on the Pollock biography and paralyzed with despair over leaving it unfinished, while Steve fought a losing battle to encourage and console me. I watched on television the scene forty-five blocks away as the ball dropped toward the new year, 1987, and I saw myself as the ball, dropping inexorably through the last seconds/months of my life.

In retrospect, I'm surprised I pulled myself together enough to go to Phil and Marlo's dinner party that cold, early January night. I didn't have much need for celebrity friends where I was going. (That's the way I was thinking then.)

This, of course, was the fateful night Charles Grodin threw down his gauntlet. "Ah, Mayo," I remember him saying when I told him their bleak prognosis. "It's a conservative institution. What do you expect from a conservative institution? Conservative answers."

"But Sloan-Kettering . . ."

"*Another* conservative institution!" he exclaimed triumphantly. "You can't take that as the final answer. There's a whole world of experimental protocols out there, people pursuing unusual things, people who aren't happy with conservative answers, people looking for other answers. No one has the last word."

"But Jerome Posner . . ."

"I don't care where you heard it. I don't care who said it. I don't care how many letters he has after his name. *No one has the last word. . . . Except you.*"

SIX

"There's Got to Be Another Way"

GARY SHIELDS WAS only twenty when he made his pilgrimage to Mayo. At a time when his friends at Missouri State University were occupied with final exams and fraternity parties (not necessarily in that order), Shields could think about only one thing: the strange pain in his groin. Still, he waited until after his exams were finished and he was home with his parents in Palm Springs, California, to have it looked at. When the doctor at the local medical center saw his scans, "he turned pale as a ghost," Shields remembers. They scheduled him for exploratory surgery the next morning, and the pathology report confirmed the worst: Shields had an advanced case of embryonal cell carcinoma. Testicular cancer.

At his parents' urging, Shields booked a seat on the first flight to the medical Mecca, Rochester, Minnesota. "Being from the Midwest," says Shields, a native Iowan, "I just assumed Mayo Brothers was *it*." Like me.

At Mayo, Shields endured a proving ground of tests and saw a phalanx of doctors, including the head of the neurology department. What they told him was not encouraging. The cancer had spread all the way up into his lungs. His insides were riddled with it. Nodules of tumor were scattered through his organs like grapes on a vine. There was no surgery that would help him, they said, or really much of anything else. They could put him on a program of chemotherapy and radiation, but even then "they didn't hold much hope for me," Shields recalls.

He returned to his parents in California "devastated." Like me.

Like me, Shields felt the am-I-dreaming dislocation of a sudden medical crisis. "Here I was, twenty years old," he recalls, "and one minute I'm at school having fraternity parties and basketball practices and football games on weekends — the college life — and the next minute I'm wondering if I'll ever see my buddies again." Nevertheless, back at the Palm Springs Medical Center, he began the grueling program of "triple" chemotherapy that the gurus at Mayo had prescribed. It wasn't the nausea or the weakness that bothered him the most, though; it was the alienation. "Everybody stays away from you. They look at you and say, 'What's wrong with him? He's only twenty, poor guy. He must be really sick.' And they don't want to be your friend. At twenty-one or twenty-two, you've got better things to do than hang around with a guy who's full of cancer."

Then one day, Shields heard about an aggressive urologist at U.C.L.A. who had just moved to California from back east. He apparently had had some success with radical surgical treatment of testicular cancer.

This is where Gary Shields and I part company.

Like Shields's parents, I assumed there was A Right Answer; and, as a patient, my job was simply to find it. That's why I flew all the way to Mayo: to find The Right Answer. That's why it was so hard for me, on my return to New York, to keep looking. I had *done* my job — I had been to the mountaintop and heard The Last Word. I was *through:* ready to take the route of least resistance, not to ask any more questions or entertain any more doubts; ready to "take my medicine" like a good patient, and, incidentally, make my funeral arrangements.

When I finally did do something, I turned around and did *the same thing again*. I sought out the preeminent doctor at the most prestigious institution around and went to get The Right Answer again, The *Last* Last Word. When it confirmed the Mayo Right Answer, it only proved what I had been telling myself all along: This was wasted effort. I already had The Right Answer. Why was I still looking?

I'm convinced that's why some people go to places like the Mayo Clinic or Memorial Sloan-Kettering in the first place. They see it as a shortcut to the best medical care and peace of mind. They think by going to the mountaintop (and there are other mountaintops), they have done everything they can. Indeed, they have gone the extra mile. "I went to Mayo," they can tell their friends with doleful bravery (or "He went to Mayo," as Gary Shields's parents told their friends). "I've seen the best. What more could anyone be expected to do?"

But not Gary Shields. For him, Mayo was just a beginning. To his parents' dismay, he went to U.C.L.A. and met with Dr. Donald Skinner. "He was a big man," Shields recalls, "six feet five inches, at least, and young, much younger than the doctors at Mayo, very compassionate and very up-front." Skinner told Shields what he already knew: that the course of chemotherapy Mayo recommended did not hold out much hope. The disease had probably spread even since his trip to Rochester. What Skinner proposed doing was a "radical node dissection" — a huge operation in which he would open Shields up "from stem to stern" and cut out every single node of cancer in his body, as many as sixty or seventy — "like trying to take all the raisins out of a loaf of raisin bread without disturbing the bread."

If some surgeon had suggested such an operation on my tumor — an operation that gave new meaning to the term "radical surgery" — I would have dismissed him/her as an adventurer or an imposter. Mayo had said it was "inoperable." That was The Last Word.

And that's exactly how Gary Shields's parents felt. "Their reaction was that Mayo said nothing could be done. What does some guy at U.C.L.A. know?" Shields recalls. "As far as they were concerned, U.C.L.A. was just a university hospital that did a lot of experimental medical treatment, but they knew the Mayo Clinic because my father had been through there, and they thought whatever Mayo said was the way it should be."

To Shields, the argument with his parents was more than just an exercise in persuasion. Because he was not yet twenty-one, they had to give their permission for any operation. The surgery with Skinner was scheduled and canceled, then scheduled and canceled again, as the debate dragged on. When Ted and Betty Shields called their son's doctor in Rochester and heard him say it was "too late for anything radical" and "the surgery is very risky and will produce no results," they dug in their heels. "The Mayo doc really put the fear of God into them," Shields remembers. "He said, 'There's nothing to do. It doesn't matter. It's going to shorten his life. It's going to *kill* him.'"

Finally, Shields forced a decision — "because my parents were just scared to death," he says, "and so was I." If they still weren't willing to sign the papers for Dr. Skinner, he told them, he would wait and sign them himself on his twenty-first birthday — which, by now, was only days away. "Look," he said, "I know this is very tough, but Mayo doesn't leave me much hope. This doctor at least is giving me an option."

An option other than death, that is.

Gary Shields (and Charles Grodin) understood what Shields's parents (and I) didn't: that *there is no right answer*. Like me, Ted and Betty Shields were still thinking of the search for the best medical care in old-fashioned terms: Find the right doctor and get the right answer —*the* right answer. To them (and to me), a second opinion was nothing more than a confirmation — "Is the answer I already have *the* right answer?" — a reassurance that the last word really is The Last Word.

When, in fact, *there is no last word*. "I tell people there are going to be no absolutes," says Dr. Dorothy White, the pulmonary specialist at Memorial Sloan-Kettering. "I tell them that in most cases there's going to be no one thing you absolutely have to do. Some people, naturally, want absolutes. They want the doctor to say this is what you have to do. You can talk all you want about informed consent, but many people are still going to say, 'How can I possibly deal with this? Tell me what to do.'"

One of the reasons there are no absolutes, of course, is that medicine is constantly changing. Just as illness is a moving target, the doctors, drugs, technologies, treatments, and procedures shooting at it are evolving arsenals. What's incurable today is curable tomorrow. What's inoperable today is operable tomorrow. From the discovery of Legionnaires' disease to the development of gene therapy, medicine is "constantly pushing ahead frontiers," says Dr. Thomas Petty, the emphysema expert at Presbyterian–St. Luke's in Denver. One recent example is the use of preoperative chemotherapy for small breast cancers. Dr. Gordon Schwartz, a breast cancer surgeon at Jefferson Medical College in Philadelphia, has achieved astonishing success by treating stage II breast cancers with the kind of chemotherapy that used to be given only following a mastectomy. As a result, among the women Dr. Schwartz has treated, almost 85 percent have been able to keep their breasts. If further research confirms Dr. Schwartz's initial results, women may have, for the first time, an option other than losing their breasts or losing their lives.

And *that* is what the search for the best medical care is really about: options. Not just getting the last word, or finding the best doctor, or confirming The Right Answer, but *developing options*. "Knowing the best heart bypass surgeon without looking into the option of angioplasty is like calling a demolition company to solve a termite problem without first contacting an exterminator," one doctor told me. By the same token, knowing which surgical oncologist does the best mastectomies is useless, even dangerous, without knowing what other breast cancer treatments are available. "While it's certainly nice to give people hope," says Dr. Jeffrey Glassroth, a pulmonary and AIDS specialist at Northwestern University, "I think my first job is really to try to make sure they understand what their options are, so that they can make a good decision."

Glassroth tells the story of a man who suffered a catastrophic respiratory failure and, after weeks on a respirator, still very ill and short of breath, came to him for a second opinion. "The hospital where he had been treated was happy to have him breathing at all," Glassroth recalls, "and they had given him a bleak prognosis": If he didn't have major surgery, he would be condemned to similar bouts of respiratory failure for the rest of his life. Glassroth gave the man a third option. "We put him on medication to lower his stomach acid, which was spraying back up into his airways, then getting dumped in the lungs and causing all these problems. He wasn't cured, but the medication lowered the risk of another catastrophic event. Today, the man works out on a StairMaster."

The search for a "second opinion" is really the search for a second *option*— or a third option or even a fourth option. One cancer specialist suggested that patients ought to develop "five or ten options," the exact number depending on such factors as the extent of the disease, the age of the patient, even "what's going on in their lives at the time." Dr. Michael Sorrell, the gastroenterologist, recommends laying out "a smorgasbord" of options (keeping in mind that one option on the table should always be no treatment at all). The point is this: No matter how many doctors have been consulted, no matter how many opinions have been collected, no matter how prestigious the doctors or the institutions rendering those opinions, in most cases the search for the best medical care isn't really finished until there are options to choose from.

Dr. Nicholas Kouchoukos, the chief cardiothoracic surgeon at the Jewish Hospital in St. Louis, remembers a woman who was brought in with congestive heart failure, deep venous disease, pulmonary emboli, and chronic immobilization. In short, "she was literally dying," says Kouchoukos. Other doctors at other hospitals had all told her the same thing: She was not a good candidate for any kind of surgical procedure. The combination of her age (fifty-one), her medical history, and her frail health had scared them off. Then she found Dr. Kouchoukos. "She was willing to go the distance to find somebody who would give her *something* to hang her hopes on," he recalls. " In her case, that meant finding someone who recognized that there was a surgical option for her." After Kouchoukos and his team removed the blood clots from the woman's lungs, "she had one of the most remarkable recoveries I've ever seen," he remembers. "This, from a patient who was literally almost dead. And now she's restored to nearly full function."

Of course, the search for the right doctor or the right hospital will often turn up options just in the normal course: This doctor wants to operate, that one wants to radiate; this doctor wants to wait, that one wants to amputate. Most doctors today, in fact, talk not in terms of absolutes but in terms of possibilities. "It's very unusual to tell somebody, you *have* to have this operation," says Dr. Martin Malawer, Tamara Enoch's surgeon. "That's what we did ten, twenty years ago. Today I say, these are the options." A doctor may offer a variety of treatment options, all under his supervision; or, depending on the option a patient chooses, he may refer the patient to another doctor. If so, the referral should be taken with the same grain of skepticism as any referral, and a search for the right doctor *for that treatment* launched. Sometimes, as in my case, a patient can spend months talking to half a dozen doctors and still have only one option. If so, then the search is not done.

Louise Enoch understood this (the way she understood everything, intuitively). She refused to believe that her daughter's only option was to live without her leg; and even then, not to live for long. Despite second, third, and fourth opinions that all agreed amputation was the only course, she persevered until finally Dr. Malawer offered a second option. Two months after she was first diagnosed, Tamara Enoch spent more than twelve and a half hours in the operating room at the Cancer Institute of the Washington Hospital Center. Dr. Malawer and a team of surgeons made an incision from her groin to her ankle, removed her entire knee joint and a third of her distal femur, and replaced them with the latest in artificial bones and joints, bypassing and rerouting arteries, avoiding nerves where possible, and redistributing muscles from the calf to the thigh around the prostheses so the rebuilt leg could bend and flex like a natural limb.

In the recovery room after the long ordeal, Louise watched over her unconscious child. The huge bandage on her leg left only the foot exposed. And it was blue. Louise called the nurse, who came and explained coolly how the blood to the foot had been cut off during the surgery and it was nothing to worry about. Then Louise felt her daughter's foot for a pulse. There was none. The nurse said that was to be expected, too. But Louise sensed "something was not right," and insisted that Dr. Malawer come and take a look at Tamara. When he arrived, he put his stethoscope on the little blue foot and listened. Nothing. Without a word, he pulled a pair of scissors from his pocket and cut off the long gauze legging. The sight of the huge, raw wound sent Louise running from the room. "It was horrible," she remembers. A few minutes later, Dr. Malawer joined her in the hall. "I don't know why," he said, "but there is no circulation going through her leg. We've got about ten or twelve hours to find out why before we have to amputate."

Louise looked him straight in the eye. "Well, then you get back in there," she said.

Fortunately, by the time they had prepped Tamara for another trip to the operating room, her pulse had returned. Her leg had swollen so badly from the surgery that circulation to the foot had been temporarily cut off. When Malawer explained this to Louise, she grabbed him by the arm in a vise-like grip and whispered, "You're a wonderful doctor."

Through Tamara's five hellish weeks of hospital recovery, she never doubted it. Through three more trips to the operating table, through days of excruciatingly painful skin and muscle grafts, Louise never left her daughter's side and never lost faith in Dr. Malawer. Then, on a visit to the hospital only a week after their return home, a routine scan appeared to show that Tamara's cancer had spread to her lungs. The oncologist recommended an exploratory thoracotomy, a procedure in which a surgeon would open up her lung and feel the tissue inside with his fingers to detect the presence of disease. Louise immediately appealed to Dr. Malawer. To her surprise, he agreed with the oncologist. "He said it should be done," Louise recalls, "even though they couldn't be sure it was metastatic disease, because Tamara's type of cancer, when it spreads, spreads to the lungs first."

To reassure her, Malawer sent Louise to the lung doctor at the Children's National Medical Center who would do the procedure. He agreed with the oncologist and Malawer that the procedure was necessary. Not satisfied, Louise herself found a doctor at George Washington University Medical Center for yet another opinion. But he, too, agreed that the procedure was "the thing to do." That was four opinions — but still only one option. "It just didn't feel right," Louise says. When she heard that Tamara would undergo a chemotherapy protocol, Rosen T-10, named after the doctor who invented it, she set out to find that doctor and get *his* opinion. On one of her many trips to the library, she looked up his name, Gerald Rosen, and found out where he worked: Memorial Sloan-Kettering in New York.

At her own expense (her insurance, through Safeway, paid for many things, but not fifth opinions, and later would not cover braces or wigs for chemotherapy), Louise took Tamara, her scans, and all her records to New York to lay before Dr. Rosen. He gave her what she was looking for: another option. "I would go with a couple of rounds of chemo," he said, "repeat the test, and then see what happens. If the nodules in her lung are still there, then you can do the surgery. If they're not, I would just keep a close eye on it with a test every few months."

Louise returned to Washington and told Tamara's doctors to cancel the surgery. "I got a lot of grief," she admits. "But Dr. Rosen turned out to be right. After they did the chemo and repeated the test, the cancer was almost gone."

Tamara never had the surgery.

A question that patients often ask is "When do I stop getting opinions? When do I have "enough"? It's a question that doctors are concerned about, too. When does the search for the best medical care become "doctor shopping"? Where is the cutoff?

The answer is simple: When you have options. Real options. Viable options. When two or more experts in the field offer differing views of what the best course of action is, that's the time to stop and make a decision. It may be necessary to seek another opinion about the relative merits of the two (or more) options on the table (a "tiebreaker," one doctor called it), but the search for additional *options*, at least, is over.

The temptation, of course, especially if the patient doesn't like the options available — no matter how numerous — is to keep looking. "What I hate to see," says Dr. Michael Sorrell, the gastro-enterologist at the University of Nebraska, "is people who devote their lives to looking, who spend whatever remaining time they have chasing a rainbow that's not there." Patients who are afraid of surgery look endlessly for a nonsurgical option; patients who want a quick, cut-and-dry solution look endlessly for a surgeon willing to operate ("Get this awful thing out of me now!"). Searches like that inevitably produce too many opinions, or too few. "I've seen patients who, when you tell them they don't need surgery, are much happier," says Tamara Enoch's Dr. Malawer. "And they will stick with that opinion because that's what they want to hear. Well, that may not be correct." On the other hand, Dr. Dorothy White, the pulmonologist at Sloan-Kettering, tells her patients "*not* to seek twenty second opinions, not to spend endless time just trying to find the answer you're looking for," and reminds them, "there are people who will die while seeking third, fourth, and fifth opinions."

There are other temptations, as well, in the headlong, sometimes desperate push to find options that are both viable *and* attractive. Dr. White complains that some patients don't give their doctors enough time before leapfrogging to the next opinion. "It takes time for doctors to gather the information that really allows them to talk to you about your prognosis," she says. "Patients need to give their doctors a chance to get whatever tests and information they need, then listen to the information, and *then* seek another opinion." I heard about a patient in Chicago whose mother stormed into the prep room just moments before he was scheduled for exploratory surgery. She had even brought along scissors to cut the plastic intravenous line before wheeling him out the door. "I didn't know if I could take the needle out of his arm," she said later. "I was afraid I might be squeamish about it." But not squeamish about telling the doctor in the room (who removed the IV rather than let her cut it) that she had found another surgeon, in New York, whom she wanted her son to see.

Unfortunately, driven by such desperation, many patients create new viable options simply by lowering the threshhold of viability, veering off into the realms of quasi medicine and out-right quackery discussed in later chapters. To avoid that temptation, Dr. Malawer told me, patients should "always look for another opinion from somebody who is at least as expert in the field as the last person they spoke to. Don't go to just anybody. You may end up with less-reliable information or, worse, somebody who will just tell you what you want to hear." In general, if there is a viable alternative treatment, it will not take twenty opinions from experts in the field, or even five, to uncover it. More research may be necessary to find the doctor or hospital with the best alternative treatment program, but more opinions from more experts will only reiterate the menu of options, not expand it.

In the end, this is what Louise Enoch was fighting for: options. When she complained that "something didn't feel right" after four doctors all recommended that her daughter undergo exploratory lung surgery, it was the sense of entrapment and helplessness, the lack of options, that frustrated her — and that she rebelled against. "I raised Tamara by myself," she says, "and I wasn't going to let anybody else make those kinds of life-and-death decisions. I heard what the doctors were saying, but the mother in me said, 'There's got to be another way.'"

And there was. Today, fifteen years after her operation, Tamara Enoch is a twenty-three-year-old college graduate in Virginia with boyfriends, a job, and long blond hair. She skis and rides bikes and vows "not to miss out on anything." Even after years of follow-up procedures to replace the prostheses as she outgrew them, the only vestiges of her brush with death are the scar on her leg ("I can't wear shorts") and the memories of those long, sad nights in the hospital bed with her mother sleeping restlessly beside her.

There was another way for Gary Shields, too. It's been twenty-five years since his brush with death; twenty-five years since the doctors at Mayo warned his parents against the operation with

Dr. Skinner. It wasn't an option, they said, it would surely kill him. Today, he is married, has a wife and a child, plays basketball and tennis, and sees his parents at least once a week, even though they've retired from the family business, which he now runs. "I tire easily," he confesses, "but I'm still here."

SEVEN

No Stone Unturned

THERE WAS ANOTHER way for me, too. There *had* to be.

That's what Charles Grodin was saying the night he threw down the gauntlet at the dinner table: There's got to be another way. There *must* be options. My job was to find them.

That same night, Steve and I decided that we would go anywhere, talk to anyone, read anything, follow any lead, turn any stone in the search for options. This was not a pledge we made lightly. Five years earlier, we had made a similar pledge when we began work on the Jackson Pollock biography. We wanted to know *everything* there was to know about this strange, gifted, self-destructive artist with two last names. We talked to everybody who had any memory of him, we devoured all the books, magazine stories, and newspaper articles we could find, then scavenged public records, archives, and private letters for any mention of him. We searched whole states looking for former friends or fellow artists or relatives so distant they didn't even know they were relatives. In the process, we turned up all kinds of extraordinary new information.

If we could do that for Jackson Pollock, why couldn't we do the same for this strange, rare, murderous tumor with the impossible name?

We started by making a list of doctors who might know something about my tumor: how it started, how it worked, how it responded, and, of course, how to get rid of it. Oncologists, neurosurgeons, radiologists, endocrinologists: I wanted to find the best in every field — the best *for my problem,* that is. I didn't care about the prestige of their hospitals or where they went to school or how many VIPs they had treated. I wasn't going to make that mistake again. I had had my fill of mountaintops and Right Answers and Last Words. All I cared about was finding doctors who had experience dealing with cases like mine who could tell me, once and for all, what my options were.

Unfortunately, it wasn't that easy.

To our astonishment, there was no place to look: no guidebook, no data bank, no resource to help us in our search for the right doctors in the right specialties. I knew I needed an oncologist, for example, but what kind? Should I talk to a vascular surgeon, a tumor surgeon, or a brain surgeon? Or all three? I was in a wilderness without paths.

I did have one advantage, though. In 1983, Steve and I had finally put our years at Harvard Law School to good use by writing a book called *The Best Lawyers in America,* a guide to the "best and brightest" in the legal profession, which we compiled by calling thousands of top attorneys around the country and asking them to vote on who they thought were "the best" in their specialties. Because it was based on peer review, *Best Lawyers* was embraced enthusiastically by the legal community, so we decided to publish a revised edition in 1987. (For subsequent editions, we hired a small team of pollsters, which allowed us to broaden the survey considerably.)

Best Lawyers was just entering its second edition when we found ourselves at the edge of another formidable, uncharted wilderness of a profession without a guide. Only this time the stakes were infinitely higher.

We started just as we had with lawyers: by calling. And calling and calling. I sat on a stool in the kitchen for hours, scribbling names and numbers, trying desperately to make myself understood by impatient secretaries and peremptory receptionists. If they couldn't sense the desperation in my voice, surely they could hear it in my mangled words. It was during these marathon phone sessions that I learned to hold my lips together with thumb and forefinger to form those elusive consonants (a trick I couldn't use in face-to-face conversation). Still, I know I must have sounded drunk or demented. And not just because of my mutinous mouth. In my desperation for answers, I grew impatient quickly, angered easily. If someone put me off or put me on hold for too long, I would explode in a sad, sputtering spectacle of indignation. "No, I *can't* wait until next month. This is a life-or-death situation. Yes, I *have* to speak to the doctor directly. Don't you understand? I'm *dying!*"

"I know, I know," said one neurosurgeon's secretary, with infuriating calm. "They're all dying."

Of course, she was right. When you work for a prominent neurosurgeon, all your patients probably *are* dying.

Every time this excruciating phonathon turned up a promising name, I was on the phone, or on the road, or my scans went express mail in my place. Between the three of us — my voice, my body, and my scans — we covered tens of thousands of miles in just a few weeks: to Australia for an expert in vascular tumors; to Sweden for a radiosurgeon; to Israel for a neurosurgeon; plus dozens of domestic destinations: New York, Pittsburgh, San Francisco, Phoenix, Houston, Dallas, Atlanta, Raleigh-Durham, Charlottesville, Columbus, Los Angeles, Boston. As my frustration mounted — along with the telephone and postage bills (bills that insurance wouldn't pay) — I kept telling myself: *Nothing I ever do will be more important than this.* Steve had a more pointed way of saying the same thing: "The only way to beat the odds is to beat them to death."

But no matter where I went or phoned or sent my scans, the answers always came back the same: tumor inoperable; radiation advised; success unlikely; prognosis bleak; good luck.

Gradually, inevitably, my search led me farther and farther from conventional wisdom and easy answers, farther and farther from the Mayos and Memorials and the conservative heart of mainstream medicine. Like Gary Shields and Louise Enoch, I, too, found a surgeon who was willing to buck the labels and operate on my "inoperable" tumor. And he wasn't in Tijuana, either; he was at Johns Hopkins, hardly a hotbed of alternative medicine. Other doctors referred to him as a "heroic" surgeon, which I understood to mean simply that he would take on cases that nobody else dared to. He was like the noble citizen who jumps into the river to save a drowning man when no one else will. His vivid description of the surgery he proposed, however, summoned up a very different image: the surgeon as Rambo, and my brain as Hamburger Hill. When I asked him over the phone about the possible neurological price of removing the tumor surgically — the loss of muscle control, or vision, or smell, or speech — he grew vague and evasive. I crossed his name off the list.

How about surgery without a knife? Not the Filipino "healer" who magically reaches into his patients' innards with his hands and pulls out the offending organ, but a technique that the Swedes developed to zap tumors using an array of radiation beams focused on a single point inside the body. Each beam is weak enough to pass through healthy tissue without damaging it, but when all the beams intersect, the resulting radioactive "heat" can kill tumor cells. This new technique, called radiosurgery, looked like a way to destroy my tumor without risking the neurological devastation of "heroic" surgery. When I found the leading expert, a Swede, I sent him my scans in a swelling of optimism. Finally, another option. A week later, he sent them back with a note: "This tumor is too big and diffuse for treatment with the gamma knife." I crossed his name off the list.

Only a few days afterward, though, I heard about another doctor in California with a gamma knife — or "light knife" as the radiosurgeons playfully called their big reactor-fed, computer-guided machines. When I talked to him on the phone, he assured me that he had treated *many* hemangiopericytomas with his "knife," and, better yet, had seen "spectacular" results. "Those kinds of tumors just melt under the gamma knife," he cooed. I had to fight the leaping in my heart when I heard that. But the fact that he claimed to have treated so many tumors like mine — "we see them all the time" — made me deeply suspicious. I didn't know everything about my strange tumor, but I did know it was exceedingly rare. Even the people who studied hemangiopericytomas didn't see them "all the time."

A few phone calls to other neurosurgeons in the area confirmed my suspicions. In an effort to pay for his big, expensive new toy, this California doctor was promising *every* patient "spectacular" results. I spoke to several doctors who had personally seen the horrific consequences: patients whose brains had "melted," but not their tumors. I crossed that name off my list.

Also in California, I found a doctor who was destroying tumors by planting radioactive "seeds" directly into the tumors: drilling little holes into the brain and slipping the seeds in like grains of sand into an oyster. Just as radiosurgery worked over space, these implants worked over time. Their low-grade radioactivity killed the surrounding tumor cells gradually, leaving healthy brain cells, theoretically, unharmed. I spoke to *the* guru of this new technique, Dr. Gerald Levin, at the promisingly-named Brain Tumor Research Center in San Francisco, and, once again, reined in my heart as I packed off my scans, and my hopes, to the city by the bay.

Barely a week later, Dr. Levin wrote back: "The tumor that

shows on your scans appears too large for implant therapy. The consensus here is that you should seek surgical debulking and then we will review your case again."

In other words, I was back where I started.

Now there was nothing left but to venture even further onto the thin ice at the edges of mainstream medicine. "There's a world of experimental things going on out there," Grodin had said. "Look at everything. Don't pooh-pooh anything."

That's more or less what Dr. Morton Silberman was thinking the first time he heard about a new, experimental lung operation that might — just might — solve his problem. Silberman had emphysema, or chronic obstructive pulmonary disease, and not as a result of smoking. It had been diagnosed at a very early age, when Silberman was a graduate student working after school in an artist's silk screen shop. "This was 1959," Silberman recalls. "The place was filled with acetone, no exhaust fans, and nobody gave a damn." For the next thirty years, while Silberman earned an international reputation first as a veterinarian, then, in a midlife career change, as a hospital administrator, his problem remained "livable." True, the disease became progressively worse and hospitalizations increasingly frequent, but it didn't prevent him from pursuing his career with workaholic fervor and reaching the top of his profession. By 1992, Silberman was assistant director of the Woodruff Health Sciences Center at Emory in Atlanta.

He was also very sick.

That year alone, he made seven trips to the hospital. Every time, doctors would put him on oxygen, test his lungs, monitor his condition, and then, when the crisis passed, take him off oxygen and send him home. But eventually the day came when they put him on oxygen and didn't take him off. The time had come to do something about his problem, they told him, something serious. He needed a lung transplant.

There was just one problem: Silberman wouldn't take a lung transplant. Not "couldn't" — "*wouldn't*." The reason? "Ethical concerns," says Silberman. The combination of the scarcity of the organs — because the criteria for transplantation are so rigorous, lungs are in the shortest supply of all donor organs — and his advanced age — no reputable lung transplant program would transplant a patient older than sixty — made the decision inevitable to Silberman. True, at fifty-nine, he was "just under the wire," but "what about all those kids out there with cystic fibrosis?" Where he had enjoyed a "very full and rich life, traveled the world, and risen to the top of two different professions," those afflicted children "had never had a chance to understand what life was all about." It just didn't seem fair for him to take a lung that could go to one of them.

Then he heard about this experimental surgery.

He was sitting in the office of Dr. Joel Cooper at Barnes Hospital in St. Louis. Silberman had already identified Cooper's transplant program as one of the best, if not *the* best, in the country. (Emory, his own institution, wasn't doing lung transplants at the time.) The experimental procedure, called volume reduction, involved deflating a major part of the upper lobes of the lungs, folding them over, and using a new suturing technique to close them up. So far, Cooper had tried it on only thirteen patients. Silberman would be number fourteen. "And none of them had been as bad off as me," Silberman recalls.

Without hesitation Silberman said, "Let's do it."

Sooner or later, anyone who sets out to turn every stone in the effort to find the best medical care will be drawn to experimental procedures. It's inevitable. Extraordinary problems demand extraordinary solutions. Patients looking that doggedly for options are, by definition, refugees from mainstream medicine. Whether it's because their condition is so rare, or because their prognosis is so bleak, or because, for whatever reason, they feel cut off from traditional solutions (as Morton Silberman did), they end up looking for hope in the realm of big risks and miraculous break-throughs, the world of experimental protocols.

What is an experimental protocol? "Protocol" is medicalese for a course of treatment, but "experimental" is harder to pin down. Purists, of course, would say it refers only to treatments that are offered as part of a controlled, scientific study testing a well-defined hypothesis. We nonscience types, however, tend to use the term in its broader sense as applying to any treatment other than the standard one. Anything that's new and unembraced. Cutting edge.

That definition scares away some patients — and attracts others. In general, the greater the perceived inadequacy of standard treatments, the more attractive experimental options look. "Most of the people who are referred to me are kind of at the end of their ropes," says Dr. Robert Brumback, the trauma surgeon from the University of Maryland, who does a lot of nonstandard, "cutting edge" orthopedic surgery, "and that's the niche I like. Send me a difficult problem. Believe me, I don't need to fix another little old lady's hip."

But what makes a particular treatment nonstandard? As Dr. Brumback implies, it's partly a matter of how common the problem is. A fractured hip is a ubiquitous injury and the treatment for it is highly standardized. But what about a rare problem, like a trachea that's being slowly squeezed shut by a major artery? Dr. Hermes Grillo, one of the world's leading tracheal surgeons, told me about a patient who was suffering from this form of gradual strangulation, a problem so rare that in his entire career as a highly specialized airway surgeon, he had seen only five cases. Even among those five, this was the first one for which Dr. Grillo was able to devise a surgical solution. The patient was cured. Was that one-of-a-kind procedure "experimental"? "I guess you could say that," Grillo concedes, "but when does it stop being experimental?" Probably, never — technically speaking. Because the problem is so rare, there can never be a "standard" treatment. The *only* way to treat it is "experimentally."

The elaborate surgery that Dr. Martin Malawer performed on Tamara Enoch is another example of a procedure that remains "experimental" largely because it's done so rarely. The other therapy available in Tamara's case—amputation—is still considered "standard" and is widely practiced, while the special orthopedic tumor surgery pioneered by Dr. Malawer is done only in a few specialized centers around the country.

Someday, however, that will probably change.

Dr. Richard Anderson, a plastic surgeon and ophthalmologist (oculoplastic surgeon) at the University of Utah, saw a patient in 1980 with a tumor called a meningioma around her optic nerve. She had been told the tumor was unresectable, not removable — "inoperable." Her vision had deteriorated to 20/100 in the affected eye. "The philosophy back then was 'There's nothing we can do about it,'" Anderson recalls, "'we just have to wait and see,' which usually meant wait until the eye had to be taken out." But rather than wait, Anderson decided to try an "experimental solution." He removed the tumor, which decompressed the nerve, and eventually brought the patient's vision back to 20/20 with full field. Today, Anderson's "experiment" is standard procedure for treating selected similar tumors.

In the same year, 1980, an eight-year-old girl was brought into the office of Dr. Philip Pizzo with a soft-tissue tumor (like mine). It had a similarly unpronounceable name, rhabdomyosarcoma, and had been diagnosed as malignant (like mine). Doctors at another hospital had already told the girl's family there was nothing they could do. "Just take her home and make her comfortable," they said. But instead, they brought her to Dr. Pizzo, a specialist in pediatric infectious diseases and pediatric hematology-oncology as well as chief of pediatrics at the National Cancer Institute of the National Institutes of Health. With all the standard treatments foreclosed as too late or ineffectual, Pizzo put the girl on a highly experimental chemotherapy program. Today, she is a law student, and the chemotherapy she received is standard treatment for soft-tissue tumors.

These are not isolated examples. Just about every "standard" procedure or treatment began as an experiment. It may not have been part of a controlled, scientific inquiry; it may have been born of necessity, like Dr. Pizzo's; or serendipity, like Dr. Anderson's. But the lineage is always the same: Today's questions beget tomorrow's answers.

The birth is not always easy, however. Dr. Joel Cooper, Martin Silberman's surgeon, remembers "the early days," when *transplants* were experimental. "They stayed that way for a long time," says Cooper, "because there was so little success with them. In twenty years, they had forty-four consecutive failures." Now, of course, transplants are considered standard treatment, and while not exactly "routine," are done at major centers across the country. And failures are the exception, not the rule.

Thirty years ago, a woman who came to a hospital with a lemon-sized tumor in her breast would have immediately undergone a mastectomy, according to Dr. Gordon Schwartz, the breast cancer surgeon at Jefferson Medical College in Philadelphia. That was standard treatment. To have done anything else would have been not just experimental, but irrational. Maybe even malpractice. "Then we learned that doing a mastectomy when the tumor is that big will only encourage the growth of smaller tumors and make the patient worse," says Dr. Schwartz. "So *twenty* years ago, she would have been diagnosed with inoperable cancer and she would have died." So what had been "experimental" became standard, and what had been "standard" became malpractice.

And what about *ten* years ago? What was "experimental" then? "We were just learning about chemotherapy," Dr. Schwartz recalls, "but it would have been considered foolhardy to try it on a tumor that big." And what about today (when that woman actually did walk into Dr. Schwartz's office)? "I explained to her about induction chemotherapy and we just melted that thing down," says Schwartz. "Then we did another mammogram and couldn't find anything there. Nothing. No tumor. So we never had to do a mastectomy."

If virtually every treatment that is standard today was once experimental, it follows that many of the "standard" treatments of tomorrow can be found among the "experimental" protocols of today. So, in a way, the medicine of the future is available right now.

In the future, for example, fewer people will be condemned to a life in darkness. Thanks in part to the experimental work of Dr. Anderson, the oculoplastic surgeon, selected tumors of the optic nerve that are now widely considered inoperable — making blindness inevitable — will be operable. Dr. Anderson treated a young boy for a glioma of the optic nerve, a congenital growth that frequently causes the eye to bulge, gradually lose vision, then go blind. "The accepted philosophy has always been that there is nothing we could do for him," says Anderson. "Until the eye went blind, when we would take the tumor out." But Anderson discovered that in some cases the impaired vision and other symptoms were caused not by the tumor itself but by fluid leaking from the tumor and putting pressure on the nerve. By going in and opening up the nerve sheath, he was able to relieve the pressure on the nerve and preserve the patient's vision. That sight-saving procedure, however, is still officially "experimental" and not accepted by many surgeons.

So is the limb-saving work of Dr. Bruce Browner, an orthopedic trauma surgeon at Hartford Hospital in Farmington, Connecticut. Dr. Browner tells the story of an insurance salesman in his late fifties who was in an automobile accident and broke his tibia (the long bone of the leg below the knee). It didn't heal and it didn't heal. For two years, the man limped around with a huge, open, bone-showing wound that wouldn't heal. After several operations failed, his doctors told him there was no option except amputation. Then he found Dr. Browner.

Browner put the man in an experimental device called a circular fixater, a series of metal hoops and wires that attaches directly to the bone and holds it in place long enough to allow new bone to grow. Because the device slowly pulls the bone apart, one millimeter a day, simulating the conditions in a child's growth plate, it literally *forces* bone growth. In addition to treating serious bone infections, it can be used to lengthen limbs and correct deformities, while giving the patient full freedom of movement.

These are just two out of hundreds of examples. "New procedures arise all the time," says Dr. Joel Cooper. Indeed, the technology changes so fast in Cooper's field, transplants, that new things sometimes become available *while a patient is waiting* for a donor organ. That was the case with Morton Silberman's experimental lung volume reduction procedure, which sacrifices the more diseased part of a patient's lung to allow the remaining portion to function better. Today, only a few years after his surgery, Morton Silberman is breathing better than he has in ten years, and Dr. Cooper's pathbreaking procedure is now performed in a number of centers, including Emory.

Farther out on the experimental frontier, there's the emerging field of xenografts — transplantations from one species to another; and, of course, the hugely important work being done in genetic and immunological therapies: manipulating the body's own formidable mechanisms in the fight against diseases of all kinds, even inherited ones. Much of it is still in the "preclinical stage," according to Dr. Pizzo at NIH — "happening in the test tube and in experimental animals" — but could be available for clinical testing before the end of the decade.

This is what Charles Grodin meant, I think, when he warned me not to pooh-pooh *anything*. What seems far-fetched today (lung

96

transplants? gene therapy?) might be Nobel fodder tomorrow. At least that's what I told myself as I slogged through medical journals with a dictionary at my side: This year's marginal note might be next year's miracle cure.

But all I found was another blind alley.

What I didn't realize, as I logged hour after mind-numbing hour with articles that might as well have been written in Sanskrit, was that most of what I was reading was already old news. There is, in fact, a delay of at least three years before experimental protocols find their way into print. That's three years from the time the protocol is *finished*— after the clinical results are in, the data have been analyzed, and *a benefit has been proved*. If the protocol deals with a rare condition, like mine, the delay can be even longer. "A conscientious doctor won't publish just on the basis of a few patients," says Dr. Nancy Ascher, the liver transplanter at the University of California at San Francisco who does truly cutting-edge experimental transplant surgery. "So you either wait until you have enough patients to publish, or you never publish. The fact is, a lot of protocols never get published."

Never get published? If the results of an experimental protocol were never published, or published only after years of delay, how could desperate patients like me, straining their eyesight into the wee hours of the morning in the medical library, ever find out about them? How, indeed, would other doctors find out about them?

The answer is: They wouldn't — unless they went to the source. "The patient's obligation is to get current information," says Dr. Cooper, who waited a year and a half before reporting his first lung transplant to journals so he could have more time to monitor his patients, "and the truly current information comes from the doctor who's doing the experimental work." In addition, almost every medical center publishes lists of the experimental protocols being conducted within its walls, and the NIH publishes lists of experimental protocols that it sponsors throughout the country.

The problem is, the doctors doing the best experimental proto-cols, like Cooper and Ascher, are the least likely to "advertise" their work, in journals or anyplace else, until the results are in. "Responsible physicians are concerned and conservative," Dr. Ascher reminded me. "They will wait until they have the data."

Others, however, are not always so conscientious.

Like the California radiosurgeon who promised to "melt my tumor away." Far from husbanding results, taking "one patient at a time," and waiting three years for journal publication, the purveyors of this "experimental" procedure put out a slick color brochure that promised "miraculous" results with a "stunning technological leap into the future" called radiosurgery. Unfortunately, such "false alarms," as Dr. Cooper calls them, are becoming more and more common as marketing invades medicine.

As an example Cooper told me about another doctor in California (why is it always California?) who advertises that his center can *cure* emphysema. How? With laser lung surgery. The laser business, if not outright quackery, seldom works as advertised, and even then not in a consistent fashion, and not without major hazards, according to Cooper. "A lot of people have been made worse." Even more troubling, though, is the doctor's financial stake in treating patients with his "miracle cure." Not only does he go out in search of emphysema patients, according to Cooper, but when he finds them, he charges the hospital $1,500 for every one he sends their way. "He makes a tremendous amount of money," says Cooper, "preying on the miseries of these patients who can't breathe and are so eager for a solution that they don't look before they leap."

One of those patients found his way to Dr. Cooper. The patient had done nothing more than respond to the center's advertise-ment by filling out an application form and sending it in. A few weeks later, someone from the laser center called to say that they had a vacancy the following Tuesday. "Why don't you come in and have your operation," they said. "But you haven't even seen me yet," the patient protested. "That doesn't matter," they said. "We'll see you when you get here for your operation."

Obviously, not every experimental protocol or cutting-edge procedure will go on to become standard practice. Some will drop away. Some will turn out to be misconceived; some will be outrun by technological advances; some will run into dead ends; some will get shut down by the authorities; some will prove impractical, some, ineffectual, and a few, dangerous.

How can someone tell the difference? How can a patient like me looking to take advantage of tomorrow's medicine today, a patient who can't afford to wait to see which experimental protocols withstand the test of time and mature into standard procedures, how can that patient tell the good from the bad?

That was exactly the question I was asking myself, over and over, as I sat in the office of Dr. Sadek Hilal and listened to him explain his new, experimental method of "shrinking" tumors like mine.

EIGHT

Stay of Execution

ON MY WAY to the huge Columbia-Presbyterian Hospital complex on the upper, upper, Upper West Side of Manhattan, I felt like a lawyer going to argue a last-ditch appeal for a condemned man — who was also me. All of Steve's and my calling and searching still had not turned up any truly viable alternatives to radiation. And no one, not even radiologists like Dr. Harrison, could work up much enthusiasm for that.

Then came word of this doctor at Columbia-Presbyterian's Neurological Institute who was developing a new method of shrinking vascular tumors like mine. He, too, was a radiologist. Indeed, he was chairman of the neuroradiology department. And he had a strange name: Sadek Hilal.

I tried hard to keep my hopes under control. I had rolled this stone up the hill too many times, only to see it slip at the last minute and tumble back into the depression where it started ("Dear Mr. Smith, the tumor is too big . . . the consensus here . . . let us know . . .") Still, I felt a needle of disappointment when I arrived at the Institute and was directed to Dr. Hilal's office *in the basement.*

My only other trip to Columbia-Presbyterian had been to visit their eminent neurosurgeon Bennett Stein, an immensely dignified, softspoken man whose big, airy office on a high floor of the Institute was crowded with diplomas and commendations and spectacular views of the Hudson River. (Stein had agreed with all the other eminent neurosurgeons that neurosurgery, eminent or otherwise, was out of the question. The risks were simply too great.)

Dr. Hilal, on the other hand, had to be some kind of nocturnal animal. The labyrinthine route to his office lay "past the furnace room, past the incinerator, past the laundry room, then take a left and go down the stairs again," according to the guard at the main entrance. And even when I followed the directions, it wasn't easy to find. The dark hall, tiled like a subway station, merely widened and brightened into a space with three or four chairs and a small sign: "Patient waiting. No smoking." Next to the sign was a small window through which I could see a nurse's cap. I walked up to the window and looked through.

Behind it was a different world. People dressed all in blue or green or white darted back and forth, pushing carts, wheeling gurneys with motionless forms under sheets. There were tubes and pipes and ducts in the ceiling and colored lines on the floor. Huge stainless-steel doors plastered with warning signs gave onto rooms filled with mammoth, whining machines or dark with computer screens. The fact that it was all happening deep underground lent the scene an eerie, almost diabolical air.

Not exactly promising.

"Dr. Hilal will see you now," the nurse said as she opened the door to this netherworld and led Steve and me to a long, narrow room lined on both sides with x-ray lightboxes. The boxes, dozens of them, were lighted but empty, casting a cold, merciless light somewhere between *2001: A Space Odyssey* and a McDonald's. A moment later, Dr. Hilal entered. He was a big man, with an olive complexion, some gray in his receding hair, a deeply creased face with saddlebag jowels, and dark, Middle Eastern eyes. Before saying a word to us, he attacked the lightboxes, thrusting sheet after sheet of x-rays into their metal clips. If one missed, he would catch it and thrust it again, even more ferociously, into place. Clearly, this was a man unaccustomed to giving the same instructions twice, even to inanimate objects.

The screens around us were almost filled with x-rays before I recognized the ghostly gray images. They were all me. I had sent Hilal copies of two complete sets of scans (CT and MRI) from Mayo and Sloan-Kettering, as well as the infamous Mayo angiogram, dozens of images altogether, and now they were all around us: the diminishing circles of axial views, the strange Halloween masks of coronal views, and the crazy, calligraphic graffiti of the angiogram, all glowing from the walls like a gallery of ghosts.

Not until the last scan was in place did Hilal turn to us. He had a jovial face, if sternly set, and a luxuriously exotic accent. "I don't think radiation is the answer for you," he began. "Look at you. You're not seventy, you're thirty-five!" I was impressed that he knew my age without checking the record. "If you were seventy and you wanted to live five more years, that would be one thing. Then I would say, fine, radiate. But you're thirty-five and you want to live another, what? *Forty* years, no?"

I nodded agreement. Forty years? No one else had been willing to commit to *four* years, much less forty.

"My point is," he continued, "we don't know what are the long term effects of radiation like this. It could damage the surrounding brain tissue. It could make the tumor you have more aggressive. It could even generate additional tumors down the road. And the longer you live, the greater the likelihood of something like that. We just don't know. We don't have the kind of longitudinal studies to predict what the effects will be, which is why I would not radiate someone your age."

Was this good news or bad? Was he saying that there was another option that would allow me to live forty more years, or was he just saying that even radiation wasn't an option — leaving me with nothing? Was he opening a new door or closing the last remaining one?

"There is another way," he said, as if reading my thoughts. He pulled from his pocket a small glass vial which he held out for our inspection. It was half-filled with a white, flaky, snow-like substance suspended in clear liquid. "It's a special silicone," he explained. "I developed it myself." He shook the little bottle and the flakes of silicone clouded the liquid (think of the "Rosebud" opening in *Citizen Kane*). "We inject this into the blood vessels feeding your tumor" — he turned to the scans behind him and pointed with great authority into the haze of imagery — "here and here and here." He brought his hand in front of his face, fingers wide, then slowly closed it to a fist. "And we *starve* the tumor."

"Do you mean you can kill it?" I asked, fighting to hide the hope in my voice.

But Hilal wasn't about to be caught in a promise he couldn't keep. "I think I can do you some positive good," he said in theatrical reserve. "We should talk in terms of reduction. I would think we could achieve a fifty to eighty percent reduction in the size of the tumor. Possibly more. Conceivably, a lot more."

What was so experimental about this procedure (called a therapeutic embolization)? It was common practice, I learned later, to embolize very vascular tumors, like mine, prior to surgically removing them as a way of minimizing bleeding (remember what happened to the unsuspecting ear doctor who inadvertently hit a geyser when he punched a hole in my eardrum). Indeed, before my brain surgery at U.C.L.A. five years earlier, my tumor had been embolized to make removal easier and neater. What was experimental about Dr. Hilal's procedure was that it didn't involve surgery. The snowy material he shot into the tumor would stay

103

there. The "starved" tumor tissue would die and, theoretically, be carried away in the bloodstream. Theoretically. In point of fact, this kind of embolization with this new material and without surgery had been tried only a few times and only by Dr. Hilal and only in this porcelain and stainless-steel underworld below the streets of Manhattan.

"What are the risks?" I asked, not really sure if I wanted to hear them.

"The primary danger, of course, is neurological damage," he said. I was impressed that he didn't flinch or avert his avuncular gaze as he moved from good news to bad. "Some of the shavings might escape and, instead of blocking the vessels to the tumor, block other vessels leading elsewhere in the brain. That could cause strokes or other kinds of damage to nearby structures like the optic nerve. I don't need to tell you that we are very careful where we put these things," he shook his little bottle again, "and we would only do as much as we can do safely. I don't want to minimize the risks, but I think you will find that they are nothing compared to the risks associated with other solutions."

Finally, I had found what I was searching for: an alternative to radiation (other than death, that is). Finally, I had an option.

Or did I?

It is almost a Newtonian law of illness that the sicker the patient, the less likely he or she is to question good news. The desperate are the beggars of hope; they can't afford to be choosy. When someone offers them a reprieve — or just a stay of execution, as Hilal offered me — their first and overwhelming reaction is gratitude, not skepticism. Unfortunately, the need to ask questions — a constant in medicine, even for conventional treatments — is nowhere more compelling than in the very area of medicine where virtually *all* patients are desperate: experimental treatments. I, for one, didn't want to know if someone else thought Dr. Hilal's new procedure wasn't scientifically sound. I didn't want to get a dispassionate assessment of the risks from another doctor. I was uncomfortable even getting Hilal's assessment of the risks, afraid that it would shake my hope. If ignorance was necessary to keep that hope alive and unshaken, I was willing to pay that price.

In fact, I could have ended up paying a much higher price.

What *should* I have done (after fighting off the urge to accept good news unquestioningly)? How could I have determined, beforehand, that Dr. Hilal's experimental procedure was scientifically sound, medically justified, and reasonably safe? How does a patient, like me, who is forced to seek treatment outside the medical mainstream, in the tricky rapids of experimental medicine, tell a good protocol from a bad one, a charlatan enterprise from a well-intentioned but faulty enterprise from a cutting-edge experimental procedure — the "standard" of tomorrow?

The answer to all the above, according to Dr. Joel Cooper, the transplant surgeon, is, "*Ask questions.*" Questions like: What institution is the protocol affiliated with? How many patients have undergone the treatment? What were their results? What was their hospital survival rate? Their one-year survival rate? How long has follow-up been done on those patients? What percentage of the patients have been tracked for follow-up? ("Twenty-five percent isn't good enough," says Cooper, who pays for his patients' plane tickets if they can't afford to come back to see him for follow-up.) How long has the treatment team been together? What did the members of that team do before teaming up? How many procedures does the team do in a year? "Don't be afraid to demand numbers," Cooper advises, numbers that should be available from the doctor, the hospital, or, for the experimental protocols they sponsor, from the National Institutes of Health.

Of course, Cooper himself is the first to admit that numbers have problems. He should know. His specialty, transplants, is perhaps the most closely monitored and thoroughly enumerated in medicine. The United Network of Organ Sharing, with support from the government, puts out center-specific data on all the transplant programs around the country, experimental and otherwise. "But you can't just look at the raw data," says Cooper. "There are all kinds of reasons why one center may have better numbers than another. Like, for instance, the difficulty of the patients they treat."

This is the other side of the coin of experimental protocols — the doctor's side. Just as the most desperately ill patients are often drawn to experimental treatments, doctors doing those experimental treatments tend to take the highest risks with the most desperately ill patients. Innovative treatments, high risks, and desperate illness may add up to exemplary, compassionate medicine, but they don't always add up to good numbers. "You have to maintain a certain level of results to be considered outstanding," says another eminent transplant surgeon, Nancy Ascher, "but that's inconsistent with doing innovative things, because you can't do ten experiments and not lose some patients."

In short, it takes a special kind of doctor to venture into experimental medicine: not just a creative, innovative one like Dr. Hilal with his Rosebud flakes, but a thoughtful, conscientious one as well, one who is capable of striking the most exquisite compromises between the injunction to do no harm and the compulsion to relieve suffering. "Experimental procedures put us as physicians and surgeons in an uneasy position," says Dr. Richard Anderson, the oculoplastic surgeon, "when we think something might work but haven't had the opportunity to prove it; when we *know* that it works and yet don't have an animal model to do research on and prove it. And, of course, many of these conditions are rare events. You haven't got a series of a thousand cases, and you aren't going to get one. It demands a special kind of doctor to press ahead under those circumstances."

For one thing, it demands a doctor who is undeterred by the

potential for lawsuits. "If you're trying to protect yourself first and take care of your patient second," says Anderson, "if you're playing that kind of game, you can't do these sorts of procedures. You have to be willing to stick your neck out and go the extra mile on an unproven or uncharted course. That, too, demands a special kind of doctor."

What it *doesn't* demand is an entrepreneur.

Unfortunately, the world of experimental medicine is shot through with them: entrepreneurial doctors who, like the California radiosurgeon who promised to melt my tumor away, have a substantial economic stake in the treatments they peddle. Desperate patients, refugees from mainstream medicine, make easy targets for extravagant promises ("spectacular results"). With the recent boom in medicine-for-profit treatments and clinics, most of the doctors I spoke to advised patients considering an experimental procedure to ask yet one more question: What is the doctor's personal financial interest in the treatment being offered?

"Medicine is a wonderful profession," says Joel Cooper, "but unfortunately, and particularly in this day and age, there's an awful lot of hype going on. It's very sad. It is promulgated by individuals who may in every other aspect appear reputable, except for the emphasis on marketing." Cooper cites the case of the laser surgeon in California who is vice president of the company that "sells" emphysema patients to hospitals. "The bottom line in these kinds of operations is that the bottom line comes first," says Cooper, "and you can't practice first-rate medicine unless the bottom line is that the *patient* comes first. The patient's interest has to come first, not the doctor's."

The best example of what Cooper means by "putting the patient first" comes from Cooper himself. When he moved his world-renowned transplant program from Toronto to the Barnes Hospital in St. Louis, Cooper went to the director of the hospital and told him, "These are the rules. I get to transplant whoever I think needs a transplant. No up-front money, no guarantees, and we do it for nothing if the patient has no resources. We do not want to have people selling their houses."

In addition to a special kind of doctor, experimental treatments also demand a special kind of patient. "This type of procedure," says Dr. Anderson, "really requires a patient who is willing to understand that you haven't tried this before and who is willing to take these risks along with you." Dr. Cooper jokes with his patients: "Does your doctor know you're here? If he does, either he thinks you're crazy, or he's a friend of mine." But patients in experimental protocols tend to talk of their choices in the same terms as their doctors — as pioneers driven by promise and sacrifice. "There is a thrill," one of Cooper's patients told me. "You're at the edge of knowledge with the brightest people." Another patient I spoke to, who participated in the early AZT protocols for people with HIV, described "the psychological advantage of feeling that you're contributing to science regardless of what the outcome might be for you individually. For me, it was a way to make some sense out of my illness, out of my death, by contributing to the understanding of this disease." Not unimportantly, that patient's doctor told me that he had almost certainly "lived longer as a result of having taken part in that protocol."

So, in addition to asking if the doctor is the right kind of doctor to be doing an experimental treatment, a patient needs to ask if he or she is the right kind of *patient*.

Was I the right kind? I certainly wasn't as well informed as I should have been. If the first duty of patients considering experimental treatments is to ask questions, then I was derelict in that duty. Nor did I feel particularly charitable. The thought that I might be advancing the scientific understanding of hemangiopericytomas did not fill me with serenity. And I certainly did not feel brave.

What I did feel was desperate. After months of resistance, I had finally given in to the urge to plot doomsday scenarios, bleaker and bleaker visions of what could go wrong: losing my sight, losing my face, losing my voice — both spoken and written — losing my . . . what was left after that? I may not have had the skepticism, the inquisitiveness, the selflessness, or the serenity of the best patients, but I did have the one thing that is truly essential for patients undertaking experimental treatments: the conviction, the unshakable conviction, that there is no other way.

And what about Dr. Hilal, that dyspeptic Egyptian deep in the bowels of Columbia-Presbyterian? Was he the right kind of doctor? Certainly he seemed the kind of doctor who "likes a challenge," to borrow a phrase from Robert Brumback, the trauma surgeon, a doctor "who prefers patients who are at the end of their rope," a doctor who likes difficult cases because they get his "motor running." The more difficult, the better. Dr. Brumback refers to himself as "the catfish of trauma. What falls to the bottom of the pond ends up in this office, and I like that position." Hilal was that way, too. He seemed to draw strength from the impossibilities of my case: the inaccessibility of the tumor, the unavailability of other treatments, the grave consequences of doing nothing, the dangers of doing anything. And his strength gave me strength. I emerged from his office after that first meeting buoyant with optimism, feeling something I hadn't felt — hadn't let myself feel — since that black Christmas months before: hope.

Perhaps the best description I ever heard of what to look for in a doctor — which applies to all doctors, but especially those with whom a patient is considering embarking on an experimental treatment — came from Dr. Peter Scardino, the urologic oncologist at Methodist Hospital in Houston. "You're looking for someone with a combination of the right training and background," he told me, "someone capable of doing anything that can be done, who has the skill and aggressive attitude to do what's called for, the discipline and experience to know what the limits are, and, finally, the judgment and wisdom to say no when those limits are reached."

To find out if Dr. Hilal fit that description, I called all the neuro-surgeons and neuroradiologists I had encountered in a decade overflowing with doctors. I made calls to M.G.H., Mayo, U.C.L.A. Medical Center, the House Clinic. I reached all the way back to Dr. Wohl at Harvard, who had been my first guide down this medical rabbit hole. There is no perfect way to pick a doctor, but some ways are definitely worse than others. The worst — and also, unfortunately, the most tempting — is to rely on the opinions of other patients. Study after study has shown that what patients think of their doctor depends heavily on the course of their illness. Patients who do poorly routinely blame their doctor (often un-fairly); just as those who do well tend to give their doctor all the credit (also often unfairly). In fact, mediocre doctors can have suc-cessful outcomes just as great doctors can have failures. The best opinions, in my experience, are those of other doctors, preferably in the same or related specialties but from other hospitals. By that standard, at least, I knew I couldn't do better than Dr. Hilal. One phrase kept coming up in my conversations with other doctors about him, a phrase I learned to listen for whenever I picked a doctor: "He wrote the book."

But what about his experimental procedure? Did it meet all the criteria for experimental treatments that I *should* have asked about but didn't? Certainly it was affiliated with a reputable institution. Hilal and his underworld team had been doing embolizations at Columbia-Presbyterian for years. They had earned the respect not only of colleagues like Dr. Stein who saw the results of their work every day, but also of other neuroradiologists and neurosurgeons around the country whom I spoke to. Indeed, Hilal's reputation was that of a bold innovator whose once-experimental techniques and materials were now "standard" in radiology departments everywhere. One other thing: Dr. Hilal clearly had no personal financial interest in the treatment he was recommending.

But what about the *numbers*? How many patients had he done? What were their results? How long had follow-up been done on those patients? What percentage of his patients had been tracked for follow-up? I didn't ask those questions at the time — and should have — but, as it turned out later, asking them wouldn't have made any difference. There were no answers. Too few patients had preceded me down this road for the numbers to have any meaning, I remember Dr. Hilal saying.

In fact, he was leading me to a place where very few people, patients or doctors, had been before. There were things I could do to ease my anxiety, to reassure myself (and my parents and Steve) — some of which I had done and some of which I hadn't. But finally, when they came to wheel me down to the dungeon for the procedure, only one thing was left to cling to. After all the questions and answers, the research and reassurances, even after all the numbers, only one thing would get me through this ordeal without the panic of second thoughts that I feared most.

As I watched the corridor ceiling lights strobe by and felt the cold air of the OR, only one thing was left, but it was enough: trust.

NINE

The Hardest Emotion

Trust.

Why did I trust Dr. Hilal? It wasn't something I set out to do. I didn't make it happen. I don't think I could have. I didn't even see it happen. One day, it was just there. It was the kind of relationship I always wanted with a doctor (what patient wouldn't?) but rarely had. And I had no idea where it came from.

I have often looked back on that procedure and thought how remarkable it was that I put myself so completely in Dr. Hilal's hands. All kinds of unanswered questions hung in the air right up to the moment they wheeled me down to that basement operating room. Some of them probably could have been answered — even by Dr. Hilal — if not definitively, at least better, with another conversation, a few more phone calls, a little more digging. But I trusted him. Other questions, of course, the key ones, didn't have answers. But I trusted him.

My situation wasn't unusual. In almost every case involving experimental treatments (or even conventional treatments), some piece or pieces of the puzzle are going to remain a mystery to the very end, no matter how long and hard a patient digs. Whether it's tumor shrinkage, neurological damage, or five-year-survival rates, some question will go unanswered; some fear unallayed; some doubt unresolved. Medicine, even mainstream medicine, is too inexact a science; the human body too subtle and elusive a subject. There's no such thing as absolute certainty — either certain success or certain failure. Just as odds can be a patient's dearest ally (knowing that 10 percent *do* survive), they can also be a patient's most implacable enemy.

In that gap where scientific certainty can never reach, in the darkness where research and preparation (the patient's or the doctor's) throw no light, the only guide, the only light, is trust between patient and doctor.

Looking back, I think the trust between Dr. Hilal and me began the day I first went to see him. As Steve and I sat in the *2001* corridor surrounded by those haunting images on the lightboxes, he carefully explained every detail of my case, as he saw it, took us on a long guided tour of the scans, detailed the experimental procedure he was recommending, reviewed the alternative treatments, their pros and cons, looked me in the eye and listed all the risks of each, including his own. At each turn in this two-hour journey, he would pause and ask in his marvelous Casbah accent, "Do you have any questions?" Then wait. "Are you sure?"

Between us, we asked a lot of questions, but when he was done, he pressed yet again, "Do you have any more questions?" and waited. We asked some more questions, but no matter how many we asked, it didn't seem to satisfy him. "I think you should go home and think about it," he said. "Then you will come back with more questions. Remember, I need your questions to know what you're thinking. Only if I know what you're thinking can we be successful partners."

Partners?

I had never heard a doctor use that word before. From the days of Carey Paul and football physicals through Dr. Heidigger and his plastic skull, I had sat in many doctors' offices, more than I cared to recall, but never saw myself as anyone's "partner." Tumor guru Jerome Posner certainly wasn't taking on any partners. At first, I thought perhaps I had heard Hilal wrong, perhaps his command of colloquial English wasn't up to his medicalese. (Too many John Wayne movies in Egypt?) But the next time I saw him, and the next, and the next, he kept harking back to it: We were "partners" in this process; I had to keep up my end of our "partnership"; partners ask questions; partners make decisions together; partners help each other over the rough spots.

I admit it came as a complete surprise to me, as I think it would to most patients, that any doctor would want to be a "partner" with his patients.

In fact, I've learned, *most* of them do.

At least, most of the best ones. Some doctors, of course, are still operating in a previous era. Like the doctor who told Joan Teckman that she had cystic fibrosis. Teckman was a nineteen-year-old nursing school student when she had *her* conversation in front of a lightbox. "I was all alone," she recalls, "a long way from home, totally away from my family, when the doctor came in and said, well, you have cystic fibrosis. It was, like, so matter-of-fact." What the doctor didn't know was that Teckman's sister had already died of CF, a pulmonary disease that is typically diagnosed in childhood. When Teckman protested that she felt fine, indeed she had been a championship swimmer all through high school, the doctor pointed at her x-rays and said, "You couldn't have been a competitive swimmer with these lungs."

"Fine," said Teckman, "have it your way. But those people who gave me the medal for the Missouri state title my freshman year are gonna be surprised." When she told the doctor that she went to nursing school, he shook his head again. "You'll have to quit and go home to be with your folks," he said. "You can't continue nursing school in your condition."

Teckman started to cry. The thought of putting her parents through the agony of CF all over again hurt far more than the death sentence that had just been handed down so cavalierly. The doctor, flustered, called a nurse and told her to contact patient psych services. "This guy wanted to send me to a shrink," Teckman recalls ruefully, "you know, like, 'This woman's losing her mind.' I thought, God, you're a jerk." Not as much of a jerk as the doctor at a Chicago-area hospital who told a patient I spoke to that he needed surgery and then, when the patient refused to give his permission until he had researched other options, threatened to have him declared incompetent so they could do the surgery *without* his permission.

The days of doctoring by diktat are over. Doctor-patient partnerships have replaced the pedestal. And most of the doctors I talked to welcome the change. "I think the relationship between the physician and the patient is now at a point where there has to be more than the old 'I'm the professor and I'm the doctor, and I'll tell you what to do,'" says Dr. Michael Zinner, chairman of surgery at Brigham & Women's Hospital in Boston. "I think both physicians and patients now expect a union of two minds coming to a conclusion, a process in which the patient has a significant involvement in the decision making. It's the difference between treating a disease and treating a patient." Dr. Andrew von Eschenbach, the urologic cancer surgeon, tells his patients, "We're going to establish this convenant of trust. But you have to remember that to have trust, you must have faith — faith that *together* we can overcome this problem." Dr. William Wood, an eminent breast cancer surgeon and chairman of surgery at Emory University Hospital in Atlanta, says, "The idea is to get patients on the team with you." Dr. Michael Sorrell, gastroenterologist at the University of Nebraska, is even more blunt with his patients, "Look," he says, "I can't do it alone."

Why are doctors — some, at least — embracing this new role? In some ways, it does make things easier for them — "psychologically easier," according to Dr. Dorothy White, the pulmonologist at Sloan-Kettering. "If you have a partner," says White, "you're no longer solely responsible for everything that happens, or doesn't happen. It's the patient's choice, too. 'I didn't do it, *we* did it.' Patients share both the decision making *and* the blame." (In reality, White concedes, most patients, especially those with serious illnesses, are heavily influenced by what their doctors tell them. "It is a very, very rare patient who, if the doctor spends the time talking and making them knowledgeable, won't follow the doctor's advice.")

In other ways, though, making the patient a partner makes a doctor's job harder — sometimes, a lot harder.

It requires listening, for example. That sounds simple, I know, but inattention from doctors is a perennial winner in patient-complaint surveys. One woman I spoke to went to see a doctor to help her decide what treatment to pursue for her advanced lung cancer. After a long meeting, she waited for his call. And waited and waited. It never came. When she called him, he said he had forgotten. "There was nothing really wrong with this doctor," she said, "he just wasn't paying attention. I figure, if you've shown a doctor that you have something potentially life-threatening, he can't just *forget*. But he did. Sometimes what looks like incompetency is really just not paying attention."

I remember going to see a doctor in New York once, a specialist in tumor-induced bone diseases like mine. I sat down and told him I had "oncogenic osteomalacia" which was caused by a "hemangiopericytoma in my right temporal lobe." I wasn't trying to be pretentious. I just thought I could save us both some time by skipping the lengthy recital of symptoms. Well. He looked at me with a skeptically arched eyebrow and muttered something terse like, "We'll just see." He then proceeded to put me through two days of examinations, tests, and scans, in a furious — and ultimately unsuccessful — effort to prove that I was *wrong*. I thought I had just stumbled onto a uniquely dysfunctional doctor until I heard similar stories from other patients: stories about doctors who, no matter what their patients told them, set out to disprove them — either to prove that, in fact, there was nothing wrong; or that it was minor and nothing to worry about; or, as in my case, that what was wrong was something else entirely. (My doctor suggested that perhaps I was anemic. Every time I tried to explain my symptoms and my long history, he would pat me annoyingly on the head, then walk out of the room.)

"I would say that half of the people who come here," says Diane Blum, the executive director of Cancer Care, a remarkable cancer patient support resource in New York, "complain that they don't get enough time, they don't get their questions answered, they don't understand, and they feel they want more. The greatest source of aggravation is communication with the doctor. One of our most popular talks around here is how to communicate with your physician."

"Somebody just sit and talk to me!" That's all Joan Teckman wanted after "that jerk" told her she had cystic fibrosis and had to quit nursing school, then walked out of the room. "I just wanted somebody to give me a little time and attention," she recalls. Finally, someone did: a resident in first rotation out of medical school. "If it wasn't for him," says Teckman, "I would have been an absolute basket case."

As the wife of a physician (who dated her husband all through his residency), Teckman understands why listening is so hard for doctors. "These guys don't even get time to go to the bathroom," she says, "but I think if they knew their patients better, they could take better care of them."

Curiously, the doctors who seem most willing to listen to their patients and explain things to them, in my experience, are the very best doctors at the upper reaches of medicine. One would think that doctors at this level of sophistication and expertise would have the least patience for questions as well as the least time for patients. In fact, as a general rule, they have the most. Or, rather, they *make* the most. "You have to see the patient, talk to the patient, really get to know the patient," says Dr. Hermes Grillo, the leading tracheal surgeon in the world. "If you spend a little time with patients, most of them will respond well to you and develop a feeling of confidence in you."

When Harold and Melissa Taylor chose Dr. Bart Barlogie out of all the doctors and hospitals they visited, half the reason was his scientific excellence, but the other half was his "genuine patient concern," according to Melissa Taylor, "a tremendous openness, a thorough willingness to inform you about the disease to the greatest possible extent, to explain to the fullest degree what the treatment program would be." Indeed, one of the things that first drew the Taylors to the faraway land of Arkansas was the fact that Dr. Barlogie "gave us as long as we wanted on the phone and didn't shy away or react in a funny way when we actually challenged him on his protocol and asked why it was better than the alternatives."

Fortunately, Joan Teckman found a doctor like that, too. Ten years after being diagnosed with cystic fibrosis (and after graduating from nursing school), she went to see Dr. Joel Cooper at Barnes Hospital in St. Louis. One of her lungs had collapsed and she needed a double lung transplant. (Because of the danger of infections, CF patients can't have just one lung transplanted.) "I had heard what a terrific reputation he had, I had heard that he was the father of lung transplants, and so I trusted the man," says Teckman. But with a reputation like that, she never expected to see much of the great man himself. In fact, while she was in the hospital, Dr. Cooper called her every night before she went to bed "to see how I was doing and if there was anything going on," Teckman recalls. When her family threw her a one-year-after-transplant anniversary party, Cooper came. Another patient of Dr. Cooper's, who was hospitalized over Christmas, received a call every day from the great man, who was vacationing with his family in Florida. "He'd make me get out of my room and come to the nurses' station to talk to him and breathe for him over the phone," she recalls. "That's what I call listening to the patient."

There is something else different about this brave new world of doctor-patient partnerships that Dr. Hilal introduced me to, something I didn't notice until after I left his office. Whether it was easier or harder on doctors, it was definitely *harder on patients*.

From the moment I found out about my brain tumor, I worried about my relationships with my doctors. After every visit to one of their offices, I was racked by second-guessing: Did I ask enough questions? Did I ask too many? Did I press too hard? Not hard enough? I treated our meetings or phone conversations like command performances, always amazed and grateful that men and women of their eminence made time for me, and nervous not to waste it; worrying afterward if I had talked too much even as I thought of all the questions I had forgotten to ask. I felt this great hunger for reassurance, a hunger that additional information both satiated and aggravated. I was equally paranoid about alienating the doctor with too many questions and missing that one key detail that would prove either the keystone to my confidence, or its utter undoing.

Dr. Hilal's repeated requests for questions swept away all that ambivalence and replaced it with a clear imperative: In a world where doctors and patients are partners, patients have not just a need, but an affirmative *duty,* a virtual requirement to ask questions. Dr. Morton Silberman, the hospital-administrator-turned-patient says, "You ought to ask questions and you ought to keep on asking them until you feel comfortable." Dr. Hermes Grillo, the tracheal surgeon, like Dr. Hilal and a lot of other top doctors, actually prefers inquisitive patients. "I like to deal with intelligent patients who ask a lot of questions," says Grillo. "They know what's going on and they know what's expected of them. I encourage questions. Questions de-mine the field."

"It's a natural human phenomenon for doctors to think more and to be more analytical when they're presented with a patient who asks questions," says Andrea Hecht, president of the Cushing's Tumor Society, who recommends that patients sit down a few days before meeting with their doctors and write out their questions. "While it's perfectly acceptable to tell the doctor that you're scared," Hecht adds, "it's important not to be hysterical." She recommends telling the doctor: "I just need to get these questions answered because this is very overwhelming to me. I have never had anything serious before. I don't know the first thing about my illness. Could you please answer these questions for me?" "What physician is not going to sit down and respond positively to a request like that," says Hecht, "I mean, unless he's a real jerk."

Unfortunately, it isn't enough just to ask questions. Those questions have to be *about* something. The duty to ask questions imposes a further duty on patients: the duty to know *what* to ask, which means knowing one's case. In the new world of doctor-patient partnerships, patients have to be far more knowledgeable than in the past. "The more you know about your disease," says Dr. Michael Sorrell, "the better you'll be able to take care of it. For some diseases, it's imperative. Diabetes, for example."

Joan Teckman even went to see Dr. Cooper operate on other patients before her lung transplant. For an entire week, she watched every operation he did, "thinking somewhere down the road that could be me on the table." Of course, not every patient has the time or the stomach for that kind of research, but there's no excuse for not doing the kind of self-education Louise Enoch did when her daughter, Tamara, was diagnosed with bone cancer. "There is so much information available at the National Cancer Institute, on-line services, or libraries," says Tamara's surgeon, Martin Malawer. "That's the first thing I would do with any serious disease, I'd go to the library. And the patients are the ones who should do it."

That's especially true with rare diseases. "The rarer the problem, the more important it is that the patient do his or her own research," says Dr. James Kirklin, the eminent heart surgeon at the University of Alabama. "Because, when you start discussing nuances with your doctors, questions will generate additional questions and, with uncommon problems, the doctors simply may not know the answers. They may not really feel confident to discuss all the potential outcomes — is there a chance of getting better spontaneously? is this getting worse? is this metastasizing? — but they may not want to acknowledge their lack of expertise." (In cases like that, I would add, patients should not only research their diseases, they should replace their doctors.)

The first step in researching any disease, common or rare, is preparing a medical history. Dr. Thomas Petty, the pulmonary and critical care specialist at Presbyterian–St. Luke's in Denver, had a patient, a thirty-four-year-old lawyer who was coughing up "large quantities of bright red blood." Recognizing that this was "not normal," he traveled from doctor to doctor, hospital to hospital, looking for an explanation. They bronchoscoped him, listened to his lungs, took scans, drew blood, and so on and so on for *ten years,* but still no one could explain why he was coughing up blood.

Finally, he ended up in Dr. Petty's office in Denver. "I sat him down and asked him to think back to the first time he ever coughed up blood," Petty recalls. "And the guy looked at me kind of strangely and said, 'Nobody ever asked me that question.'" He proceeded to tell Petty about the time when, as a sixteen-year-old, he was called into the principal's office to answer for a prank. When the principal started reprimanding him, he got "this warm, funny feeling" in his mouth, and when he opened his mouth, out came blood.

Then there was the time, after he became a lawyer, when he was having a real battle with an opposing attorney in court, getting angrier and angrier, until suddenly he had that feeling again. Sure enough, he opened up his mouth and out came blood. Then there was the most recent episode. Only days after buying a new car, he turned the key and it wouldn't start. A brand-new car. He was furious. And then he got that feeling in his mouth again.

Just from the patient's story, Petty was able to deduce that blood was leaking from his bronchial arteries into his lungs when his blood pressure rose high enough. A subsequent bronchial angiogram proved Petty was right: There were weak spots in the walls of the bronchial arteries. The reason nobody else had discovered them in *ten years* of looking, says Petty, was that "no one had ever sat him down and taken a careful medical history." (Petty's solution was to stop the bleeding by embolizing the weak arteries, thereby plugging them up. It worked. Eight years later, the man sends Petty a card every Christmas.)

To avoid just that kind of problem, I prepared a thirty-one-page "medical profile" that included a case history, a list of the doctors I had consulted (forty-two in all), a chronology of "imaging studies" (x-ray, CT, MRI, angiogram, etc.), operative reports from my various procedures, and copies of all the important correspondence from my primary doctors. (The first line of my profile: "It began with pain in my feet.") I know a breast cancer patient with an especially convoluted history who had her primary care doctor write up her history. "That way," her husband explained, "every time she sees a new specialist, she doesn't have to repeat the same story and then worry if she's left something out."

The other "duty" of patients in doctor-patient partnerships is the duty to cooperate. Before Dr. Hilal, I had always had a cordial if somewhat formal relationship with my doctors. Growing up, I was taught that they were figures to be respected — well-educated and typically well-off, upstanding, golf-playing members of the community. Of course, I also dreaded going to see them. Because pain was almost inevitably involved, the less I saw of them the better. I wasn't exactly hostile, just intimidated.

As years passed, this childhood confusion turned into a full-fledged adult ambivalence. On the one hand, I prided myself on having, in general, good rapport with my doctors. I always tried to be cooperative and pleasant, even if they kept me waiting unnecessarily or didn't give my complaints what I considered sufficient attention. On the other hand, I often worried that perhaps I was being too cooperative, too pleasant. Maybe if I pushed a little harder, was a little more demanding and a little less intimidated, I would get more attention, or better attention. For example, I wouldn't have let that foot doctor get away with telling me that I had the feet of a pregnant woman.

After the discovery of the brain tumor, when the stakes went way up, my ambivalence turned to angst. I constantly worried about whether I was making the best use of my doctors. Was I taking full advantage of them, or alienating them? Being too respectful, or not demanding enough?

This is not an easy line to walk. The slopes on both sides are slippery: on the one hand, complacency; on the other, outright hostility. Like the hostility of one patient I talked to who had been through a trying medical ordeal with her son. "I'm not particularly fond of doctors," she told me, "and I don't take any nonsense from them. They're not God. It's a wonderful profession if you need them, but so overrated."

Everyone I spoke to agreed on the need to keep that kind of anger out of patient-doctor partnerships. "It's human nature to try to be nice to nice people," cautions Dr. Kirklin. "And anybody you have to grit your teeth over is almost assuredly not going to be treated with the attention somebody else would be." I heard about one case where a patient did a lot of "acting out physically and verbally," according to the patient's doctor, "making it very unpleasant to deal with her." So unpleasant, in fact, that the nurses on the floor refused to answer her call light. "That is not the way nurses are supposed to care for patients," the doctor agreed, "but it's not just nurses. Doctors, too, have difficulty addressing a patient's illness without taking the patient's behavior toward them personally."

Does that mean that patients should be afraid to disagree with their doctors? Afraid to press them for explanations for fear that their painkiller might get delayed or their IV bag might not get changed? Not at all, says Kirklin. "If the patient just says, 'You're wrong,' or 'I want another opinion, because I don't believe you,' that would alienate the doctor. But if the patient says, 'Let's not stop here. Is there any possibility of any therapy that you haven't mentioned that could possibly help? I'm willing to try anything,' the physician can review other treatments and explain why he doesn't think the patient is a good candidate for them." In other words, disagreeing is fine — as long as it's done in an agreeable way.

Because doctor-patient partnerships place so many new demands on patients — ask questions, know your case, cooperate — some patients, like some doctors, prefer the old days. When I asked one patient why he had chosen a risky experimental chemotherapy protocol, he told me, "I just went along for the ride. I didn't look at anything, I didn't bother with anything. You can't make all those decisions for yourself. It's a time to just sit back and enjoy yourself and let other people do the work." Early in his treatment, when he went in to get the results of a test for brain cancer, that patient had told his doctor: "I want to know everything about this thing, *except I don't want to know if I have cancer or not.*" Why? the doctor asked. "Because my father can't handle it," the man said. The doctor respected his patient's request and withheld the bad news. Three weeks later, the man's mother finally told him, although by then he had already guessed.

A lot of patients, I think, are tempted to do the same, to stick their fingers in their ears, hope for the best, and put themselves entirely in their doctors' hands. With the world crumbling around them, they "don't want to bother with anything"; they just want to let go of "earthly cares" and let other people do the hard work of decision making. "From the time you're a child, you're taught that doctors have tremendous education. You learn to trust your doctor and not to question him," says Sara Glassner. "If you're sick, there's almost always an element of fear, and you want to believe, you *need* to believe, that the doctor can make you better. There are people who assume that doctors are the experts, they don't want to have to pay attention to what's happening, they don't want to ask questions. They opt for a kind of a blind faith, and that's not good. The people who do best enter into a partnership where they assume some of the responsibility for their care, where they're active learners and active participants."

Sara Glassner ought to know. Her husband, Steve, was diagnosed in 1978 with acute asthma, an extremely serious, potentially lethal pulmonary affliction. He was twenty-seven, exactly my age in 1978, and Sara was pregnant with their first child. Sara was just like thousands of wives and husbands, mothers and fathers, sisters and brothers of people who confront life-threatening medical crises, except for one thing: Sara Glassner was also a nurse.

"In the beginning, I was just like any other wife," Sara told me, "afraid because my husband was critically ill. It didn't matter that I had the knowledge and training of a nurse. I was still afraid. I went through a process like grief: being angry, denying it all, crying a lot, and then coming to some kind of resolution." Slowly but inexorably, Steve's and Sara's life was invaded by the disease. Steve was first rushed to the hospital and put on an artificial respirator (intubated) in 1982. "It was pretty frightening," he recalls, "breathing became the most difficult thing anybody could ever imagine. You've never worked so hard in your life, just to breathe."

Seeing her husband struggling for breath, Sara Glassner vowed to devote her medical expertise to his illness. When Steve was released from the hospital, Sara took over the job of monitoring his medicine and his symptoms. Steve went back to his active life of swimming and playing racquetball and working at Baker

Furniture in Chicago, as if nothing had happened. "I was a little bit cocky," he recalls. "I was young. My attitude was, 'This isn't going to happen again.'"

But it did. Only a few years later, Steve had another acute anoxic attack at home. He was battling for every breath. Sara knew he was in trouble and wanted to rush him to the hospital, but Steve resisted. "He was pretty much denying that he was in trouble," Sara remembers, "and continuing to want to manage himself at home." Finally, after a long, fierce argument, Sara put her foot down. "We're going to the emergency room!" she shouted as her husband gasped for air.

Then, on the way to the hospital, he arrested. Starved for oxygen, his heart stopped beating.

Sara managed to reach the emergency room in time for the doctors to revive him, and, after a long intubation, he was released again. But she had learned her lesson. "I realized that Steve had become too dependent on me and my medical knowledge," she says. "I made the mistake of trying to manage everything myself." He didn't know enough about his disease to know when he was really in trouble. He had left that to her. "It was then I realized I couldn't be in charge," says Sara, "*I* couldn't be in control. *He* had to be."

Patients have to be their own "case managers," says Glassner. "They need to *own their own problem,* and they need to accept responsibility for their care. When you have an illness, especially a chronic illness, you can't absolve yourself of responsibility. You can't just say, 'Well, the doctor's the one who's in charge, and he's going to do it all.' You *have* to participate. You *have* to be active." Like Dr. Sorrell, Glassner cites the example of diabetics. If diabetics understand their disease, if they learn how their disease works, how to manage their medications, and how to adjust their diets appropriately, "they can function at a higher level," says Glassner. "If they're dependent on someone else to check their blood sugar, if they just eat what they're given, if they don't understand what to do and what not to do, then they're not functioning at their highest level."

There are times, of course, when a patient needs someone else to act as case manager, Glassner concedes. "Sometimes that can be the nurse, sometimes it needs to be the spouse. For example, in my husband's case, if he's on a ventilator, he can't do things for himself. I have to do them for him." Joan Teckman, the woman with cystic fibrosis who had a double lung transplant, agrees: There are times when the patient, for his or her own good, needs to let go. "Ever since my transplant," says Teckman, "I've talked to a lot of people that have asked ten thousand questions, down to every single thing they want to know, every single thing that's going to happen. And they can turn themselves into nervous wrecks. I think the patient can *overmanage* his or her case. And in so doing, you can make yourself sicker."

Ask questions, but don't pester. Cooperate, but don't capitulate. Be your own case manager, but don't overmanage. How is a patient supposed to navigate through so many conflicting imperatives when it comes to dealing with doctors? The best answer to that question I ever heard — the best description of how to walk the fine line between deference and defiance, between pushing too hard and not pushing hard enough — came from Melissa Taylor. "Make sure that you understand what is going on," she said. "Make sure that you are not railroaded by the doctors. Don't be passive. Don't just accept what you are told. Don't just let the doctor roll over you with things that you can't understand. Ask the questions. Make sure not that you challenge what you are told, but that you question it. Make sure, even if it takes all day, that you go on asking the questions until you understand the answers to the best of your ability. There may be aspects of the problem that you will never understand, but keep on questioning until they have made you happy in your own mind."

So if these new partnerships between doctors and patients are harder on doctors *and* harder on patients, why do more and more doctors, as well as more and more patients—like me—prefer them to the old way?

Simple. Because out of these partnerships comes trust.

Not the old kind of trust, a blind faith — "Take me, Doc, I'm all yours" — based on paternalism and ignorance; but a new, more genuine, more resilient, more enduring, more beneficial kind of trust. The kind of trust that comes from *mutual* respect and communication. The kind of trust I felt with Dr. Hilal. The kind of trust that makes miracles happen. "You just keep thinking, 'Well, you're either going to die or you're going to come through it,'" said a patient I spoke to, a fifty-year-old woman who was on the brink of death because of blood clots in her lungs. "I knew I had good doctors, and I knew that they cared, and I knew they were working for me, and that means an awful lot. It really does." Another patient told me that her doctor's confidence gave her confidence; his courage gave her courage. "If you have a patient who is unwilling to give up," says Dr. Richard Anderson, the oculoplastic surgeon, "and a doctor who is unwilling to give up, there is immediately a bond of trust between them" — a bond that is harder to break than any mortal coil.

The bottom line is simply this: Patients do much better where there is trust, "when they have confidence that their care-giving team cares whether they get better or not," says Dr. Michael Sorrell. At the University of Nebraska, Sorrell regularly reminds his house staff that "there's nothing quite as frightening as being sick and thinking your doctor doesn't care if you get better or not. There is nothing more frightening than that." And there is nothing more reassuring than trusting that your doctor will do everything humanly possible to make you better. "I think sometimes we lose sight of how important the physician is in that interpersonal relationship we call trust," says Dr. Andrew von Eschenbach. "Out of trust comes that sense of hope, that faith in a positive outcome, and that sense of compassion that imbues patients with that crucial extra measure of strength."

Don't believe it? Just ask Joan Teckman.

After her sixteen-hour double lung transplant surgery, Teckman lingered on a heart-lung bypass machine "probably longer than is compatible with life," she recalls. Then her kidneys failed, and she went on dialysis for two months. "Pretty much everything that could go wrong did go wrong," she says. After three weeks on a ventilator, she had to relearn how to breathe, and how to walk, and how to eat. "But all along, I understood what Dr. Cooper was doing, and I trusted him. I trusted the people I was with." Today, Joan Teckman is swimming again. In 1993, she competed in the transplant Olympics and won three gold medals. In 1994, she married. "Every year I have is a year I never had before," she says, "and a year that Dr. Cooper gave me."

Still don't believe it?

Just ask me.

TEN

"Tick, Tick, Tick . . ."

TRUST OR NO trust, I went into the embolization procedure in March 1987 absolutely terrified. Far more terrified than I had been for the big brain surgery six years before. Why? Because I would be awake for this one. (Those whom the gods would make mad, they first make conscious.) For the craniotomy, they had put me under — way under. It all happened in the dark. I woke up sore and woozy and dying for a drink of water, but without so much as a bad dream from the operation. And, of course, knowing I would be out for the main event made the anticipation a lot easier. The only thing to worry about was that I might go under and never come back up. But that would be like dying in my sleep, which is the way everybody wants to go anyway — although not at thirty-five.

The embolization, on the other hand, had to be done while I was conscious. Because of the danger of neurological damage at every turn — from the catheter, from the dye, from the silicone "snowflakes" — they needed me awake and responsive. Every two or three minutes, some subaltern would stick his face in my face and ask, "What's your name?" or "Do you know where you are?" or "Who is President of the United States?" From the answers to these questions, apparently, they could reassure themselves that my brain was still functioning normally.

As they rolled me into the OR, the Valium had already begun to have an effect — although not enough of one. Not enough to blot out the memory of that disastrous angiogram at Mayo, the one that still ranked as the most painful and humiliating hospital experience of my life. After all, what was this experimental embolization but just another angiogram, only longer and riskier and scarier? It started off the same way, with a puncture in the femoral artery ("You'll feel a little pressure . . .") perilously near that most sensitive of regions, followed by the long, laborious process of snaking the catheter up from the groin, through the arteries of the chest and neck.

Dr. Hilal did what he could to calm me down. He explained everything as it happened, told me what would happen next and how long it would take (I found the latter especially helpful). But it was mostly just the familiar sound of his deep, accented voice, guileless and self-assured, that reassured me. It did strike me as odd, though, that a patient should be conversing with his doctor *during* the operation — asking questions, seeking reassurance. I wondered if he, like me, would have preferred me to be unconscious.

I had known doctors like that. When they brought me into the operating room at U.C.L.A. for the big brain surgery, I was heavily sedated but still awake enough to follow what was happening around me before they put the anesthesia mask over my nose and mouth. At one point, I asked one of the surgeons hovering over me to identify a big piece of equipment that a nurse was rolling into place. He looked down at me with a startled expression, as if I had spoken from the grave. "What's this patient doing awake?" he demanded in a tone somewhere between anger and astonishment.

He seemed genuinely, deeply disconcerted at the idea of interacting with the person whose head he was about to open.

But Dr. Hilal wasn't like that. He spoke to me just as if I were sitting in the chair in his office, reviewing scans, weighing options. The calmness and familiarity of that voice did more to quiet my anxieties than all the Valium in Hollywood.

Still, lying motionless on that hard table, strapped down at the wrists and ankles, drugged senseless in every part of my body except the one that mattered, my mind, I longed for unconsciousness. Why didn't I just do the damn surgery? I heard my befuddled brain ask. This wasn't medicine, this was some exotic form of torture. They even made me *watch!* Just a few feet above the table, angled so that I couldn't avoid seeing it, was a monitor that showed the fluoroscopic image of my chest, a sort of x-ray come to life. I could see the fluttering ghost of my heart, the faint, gray path of arteries, and there, making its way tentatively upstream in fits and starts, was the end of the catheter. When it made a quick move, I fancied that I felt it somewhere deep inside where I had never felt anything moving before. Now and then, a little white dye would bleed from the end to light the path ahead and I would feel a flare of iodine heat as though someone had struck a match in my heart.

When the catheter reached the arteries in my head, that's when the real torture began. In order to know exactly where to place the silicone flakes, Hilal needed a precise map of all the blood vessels around the tumor. That meant injection after injection of dye as the camera whirred and spun its image onto a computer screen for him to study. Each injection involved carefully manipulating the catheter (which could only be controlled from the distant opening in the femoral artery) into position in just the right vessel out of dozens of possibilities, then waiting while the mechanical injector coughed and wheezed and finally spit just the precise amount of dye through the catheter.

The panting of that injector was my signal. That's when I braced for the pain.

The iodine dye entered the bloodstream like a river of fire. People asked me later to describe the pain and I said it was as if someone stuck a lighted torch in your face. Imagine the worst toothache or migraine or sinus infection you've ever had, multiply it by ten, then set it on fire. Unlike toothaches and migraines, of course, this pain flashed white hot for a few seconds, then faded. But before it was gone, I would hear the whirring again, that awful whirring, and clench my fists just in time for the next fireball. And the next, and the next. For two hours.

This, of course, was exactly what I had feared most: pain. It wasn't fear of failure, or even fear of the unknown, that had made me dread this procedure so fiercely, that had kept me up the whole night before despite the sleeping pills. It was fear of precisely and only this: pain.

As anyone who has felt it knows, pain is both a powerful motivator and a powerful disabler, a powerful incentive as well as a powerful deterrent. I have no doubt that many critical procedures and treatments have been delayed or foregone for fear of it.

But there is pain and there is pain. The pain I felt lying there on the table was bad, no doubt about it. But it was nothing like the pain I would have felt if I hadn't trusted Dr. Hilal: trusted that he was doing the right thing for me; trusted that he wouldn't put me through that pain unless he absolutely had to; trusted that he cared about the outcome and making sure it justified the pain. There's no pain worse than pain without trust, the pain you feel when you think no one cares. Dr. Sorrell definitely got it right: "There's nothing quite as frightening as being sick and thinking your doctor doesn't care if you get better or not. There is nothing more frightening than that." Amen. Pain is bad. But the combination of fear and pain can be overwhelming.

I know because I've felt that kind of pain, too.

There was another angiogram — I won't say where — but it was after this one (Dr. Hilal had retired). I had weathered the storm of the procedure itself and they had wheeled me into the recovery room, which is where I encountered "The Clamp."

Because the angiogram procedure uses a relatively large catheter, it requires a fairly large puncture hole (much larger than for, say, drawing blood) and because that hole stays open for hours, the artery typically takes a long time to close back up. During that time, it's important to keep pressure on the puncture site so that arterial blood, which is under high pressure, doesn't blow through the healing hole and flood the surrounding tissue, creating a hematoma (medicalese for an area of bleeding under the skin).

Always before, when I came out of an angiogram, the doctor or one of his assistants had applied pressure to the hole in the artery where the catheter had been inserted by pressing on it with his hand. The pressure had to be firm, and, given the sensitivity of the area, was acutely uncomfortable. It also had to be applied for quite a while — half an hour or more — after which time the recovery room staff would wrap the area in a very tight pressure bandage that might stay on for anywhere from four to eight hours and I was confined to bed, immobilized, for another twenty hours. That was the drill, with minor variations, that had been followed by all six of my previous radiologists.

But not Dr. Chu.

She couldn't be bothered with anything as personal as using her hand to apply pressure. Instead, as soon as I was in the recovery room, she pulled out an elbow of shiny metal. "This is a clamp," she explained in her clipped, precise English. "We will use it to keep pressure on the insertion site." The clamp worked like a vise —*exactly* like a vise. She fastened one end to the gurney so that the other, curved, end extended out over my groin. Then she began tightening it. Each time she turned the screw, the metal arm pressed harder and harder, deeper and deeper into that softest and most sensitive of regions. Again and again she turned the screw. Harder and harder the clamp bore down. Deeper and deeper. The pain was dull at first, then sharp, then piercing. After each turn of the screw, I thought surely she was finished. The clamp couldn't be any tighter. I squirmed in discomfort to let her know that, but she ignored me and tightened it again. Finally, through the haze of sedatives, in genuine agony by now, I cried out, "It's too tight!"

She brushed my pain aside. "It has to be tight," she said brusquely as she tightened it yet again.

"Why can't you use your hand?" I pleaded.

"Sorry," she said, without a trace of real regret. "This is the way we do it. This is best. It's no different from the hand."

Only someone with a mechanical heart could think this mechanical hand was equivalent to human touch. Like most patients, I think, I can tolerate a lot more discomfort, a lot more pain, if I know a concerned, compassionate warm body is at the other end of that pain, especially a warm body that I trust. When I was a boy, my mother used to treat all my cuts and scrapes with Mercurochrome, a vile, orangish liquid (also iodine based) that, no matter how much she blew on it, always burned like crazy, inflicting far more pain than the injury itself. That was how I got through the torture with Dr. Hilal. I knew that he wouldn't be inflicting that pain if there was another, less painful way to help me. I clung to that thought even as the blowtorch of dye burned every other thought out of my head.

But Dr. Chu was different. Indifferent. The more I squirmed and cried out in agony the more firm and stoic she became — as if indifference to my pain was the truest test of her professionalism.

In twenty years of fighting cancer, through two brain surgeries, hundreds of often excruciating tests, months of hospitalization, and years of recovery, that was without doubt the worst pain I ever felt.

After the trial by fire of the angiogram, Dr. Hilal's "experimental" embolization proved anticlimactic. No whirring, no clenching, no blowtorch. Once again, I fancied I felt the soft flakes as they shot from the end of the catheter. They felt cool by comparison to the scalding dye, and one last time I pictured the scene from *Citizen Kane* as the fake snow turns to real snow and settles gently on the landscape of memory.

And the results?

"Good news and bad news," said Dr. Hilal when he came to visit me later that day in my hospital room. The good news I already knew: There had been no noticeable neurological damage from the procedure. My vision was intact, along with my speech (such as it was), my sense of smell, and my memory, all of which could have been affected. The bad news? He hadn't been able to embolize all of the tumor. There were some vessels that appeared on the angiogram to feed both the tumor and the optic nerve; to embolize them would have put my eyesight at risk, so he had decided on the spot to leave them alone.

How much of the tumor did he get? It would be at least a few weeks before we knew for sure, he said. It would take that long for the blood-starved parts of the tumor to shrivel up and die. "But if I had to guess right now, I would say fifty to sixty percent reduction."

Sitting on the side of my bed, his saddlebag jowels drooping from exhaustion or worry or both, Hilal seemed genuinely disappointed. So disappointed that I found myself trying to cheer him up. "That's pretty good," I said, still with my deflated *p*. In fact, before the procedure, he had told me "fifty to eighty percent," and I, of course, had fixed my hopes on the upper end of that range. But that wasn't his fault. Unlike the neurosurgeon at U.C.L.A. who virtually promised to "get it all out" and, even after the operation, insisted that he had succeeded, Hilal had never misled me. He had, in fact, prepared me for what he called a "partial victory." Especially in experimental treatments, he would say, results are harder to predict because predictions are based on more limited experience, "so we often have to be happy with partial victories."

I reminded him of that, then added something else he always used to tell me: "All we need is a few more partial victories, and we'll have a whole one."

Every morning for the next month, I would wake up and run through a routine of "tests" to see if the embolization had loosened the tumor's grip on my life: I tried whistling, winking, puckering, making faces in the mirror, drinking out of a glass without dribbling, holding water in my mouth without leaking, repeating "Peter Piper picked a peck of pickled peppers" — all things that I hadn't been able to do since that fateful Christmas party.

For a month, nothing. The tests left me feeling more depressed and pathetic than ever. I called Dr. Hilal, partly to ventilate my frustration and partly to drink in his encouragement. "Not to worry," he would say with fierce enthusiasm. "It will come. It will come."

And it did. One morning, at the end of the first month, I woke up and went to take my first round of pills. Still groggy with sleep, I didn't think to hold my lip against the glass the way I had learned to keep from dribbling water down my chin. Only there was no dribble. After that, not a day went by that I didn't notice something different. Little by little, my old life was coming back to me as the paralysis ebbed. I stopped taping my eye shut at night; I even stopped holding my lips together to form those elusive consonants.

I could talk again.

Dr. Hilal confirmed in black and white what I already knew in color. Scans showed that the tumor had shrunk, as he guessed, by 50 to 60 percent. I didn't care about the percentages, though. I had my life back. The crisis was past.

Like a lot of patients who win "partial victories," I was desperate to get back to my life, to put doctors and hospitals and tests and procedures and life-and-death decisions behind me, and live like all the "normal" people, the tumorless crowd that I used to envy as they passed me on the street. Fortunately, Dr. Hilal wouldn't let me get away with that. "The tumor has not gone away, you know," he would say in a mock-chastising tone, pointing his big finger at my head, the head he knew so intimately. "It's still in there and it's still growing and you need to keep an eye on it. You don't want any more surprises."

I credit Dr. Hilal not only with giving me my life back, but also with helping me keep it. If it hadn't been for him, I probably would have floated through the next few years on a cloud of denial, drawing false reassurance from my lack of symptoms — until the next, even more devastating Christmas debacle. But now I had a "partner" in my medical journey, a big Egyptian one, and he wasn't about to let me stick my head in the sand. "One benefit of a doctor-patient 'partnership,'" says Dr. Dorothy White, "is that unlike a one-time, arms-length encounter, a partnership creates obligations that survive the acute phase of an illness — obligations both ways." For my part, I trekked up to Columbia-Presbyterian every three months for scans and tests to trace the tumor's progress. Dr. Hilal's part, as he himself described it, was "to never let up on the search for a better treatment."

Only a year later, on a routine visit to his dungeon office, he told me he had found one.

The treatment he recommended was another experimental embolization, this time using alcohol instead of silicone flakes. Unlike the silicone, which worked by physically obstructing blood vessels and slowly starving the tumor, the alcohol killed tumor cells directly. So, theoretically, it wasn't necessary to embolize every vessel leading to the tumor (what he'd been unable to do in the first procedure); with alcohol, a few good "shots," so to speak, might just poison the whole tumor. That's what it had done in rats — the only previous beneficiaries of this new and untested treatment — and, theoretically, it should work the same way in a thirty-six-year-old writer. *Theoretically.*

True to form, Dr. Hilal did not shy away from detailing the risks. Just as in the silicone embolization, there was a danger that the injected alcohol might "transgress the boundaries of the tumor." No matter how carefully the catheter was placed, alcohol might actually pass *through* the tumor and end up somewhere downstream in healthy tissue. Indeed, some of the experimental rats had died from damage to the parts of their brains that controlled involuntary functions like breathing and heartbeat. Because of different circulatory patterns in rats and writers, Hilal assured me, I didn't need to worry about that, but he couldn't discount the possibility of some kind of damage.

I asked him what he would do if the decision were his. Without hesitation, he said he would do it. There was a real chance of not just reducing the tumor, but eliminating it altogether, he said, and that chance made the risks worth taking.

That was good enough for me. In April 1988, I found myself once again in the frigid underground OR at the Neurological Institute, clenching and grimacing through another round of fiery injections, clinging to my trust in Dr. Hilal and my hope, never expressed out loud, that this might just be the last time I had to do battle with this tenacious tumor.

But it wasn't to be. To Dr. Hilal's utter astonishment, the alcohol did *absolutely nothing.* Not even minimal shrinkage was discernible on postoperative scans. He scanned and scanned, then waited and scanned some more, sure that some change would show up sooner or later. But it never did. The only thing I had to show for my day of agony, besides yet another set of bad memories, was yet another affliction: Horner's syndrome.

As Hilal feared, some of the alcohol had leaked out and damaged a tiny nerve that threads its way improbably from the chest up to the eye. As a result of the damage to just that one nerve, my right eye didn't tear properly, my eyelid drooped, and the pupil in that eye wouldn't dilate fully. In addition, strangely, that side of my face didn't sweat as much as it used to — indeed, hardly sweated at all. I could be dripping perspiration off the left side of my forehead and dry as a bone on the right. This bizarre sampler of symptoms is called Horner's syndrome.

True, this was hardly the kind of grievous neurological injury that Hilal had warned me about and I had assumed the risk of, but it caused me grief nonetheless. Coming on top of the lingering deficits from surgery, the residual weakness from months of paralysis, and the self-consciousness that both those had ingrained in me, this new affliction went far deeper than cosmetics. It seemed like yet one more way in which I would never be the person I used to be. I had come through not being able to talk right, drink right, kiss right, wink right. Now I couldn't even cry right.

Of course, I realized that neither the failure of the alcohol embolization nor the neurological damage that resulted from it was Dr. Hilal's fault. That was another of the legacies of our partnership. "When the relationship between physician and patient passes the old kind of 'I'm the doctor, and I'll tell you what to do,' and reaches the point where it's really a union of two minds coming to a conclusion," says Dr. Michael Zinner, the surgeon at Brigham & Women's, "that not only allows the patient to feel like they have some control of a process that they could easily lose control of, it also means that, if they make the wrong choice, at least it's the choice *they* made, and it's their life."

It was in this spirit of a "union of two minds" that Dr. Hilal sat down with me some weeks after the second embolization to discuss the next step. What were my treatment options? In his calming baritone, he methodically laid them out: another embolization like the first one; another major surgery of some kind, conventional or heroic; radiation, either the conventional kind that Mayo had half-heartedly recommended or something more avant garde like radiosurgery or seed implantation; and, finally, nothing — just wait and see.

All the treatments on his list involved risk, he went on to say; indeed, some, like heroic surgery, involved substantial risk. Even the last option, doing nothing, was not without risk. The tumor was still there and still growing unpredictably. If it grew in certain directions — toward the brain stem, for example — it could interfere with vital functions and pose a serious, even mortal danger. In another direction, it could threaten the optic nerve and my eyesight. In another direction, it could invade the cavernous sinus, an especially sensitive nerve center at the base of the brain. If it grew in any of these directions, it could quickly turn into an urgent problem that demanded drastic, immediate action. On the other hand, it could grow in any one of several other directions and pose little or no threat at all. But it was impossible to know — or even guess — which way it would turn, or when. In short, I was sitting on a time bomb that might not be ticking now, but could start at any moment.

Together, we decided that the best thing to do was wait and watch, or, as Dr. Hilal put it so eloquently in his movie-cowboy English: "If it ain't broke, don't fix it." I would continue coming to Columbia-Presbyterian for regular scans. He would carefully follow the progress of the tumor, comparing each new set of scans to the previous ones to catch the first signs of movement, the first suggestion of direction — the first sound of ticking. The moment the tumor started to move in the wrong direction . . .

We would make that decision when the time came.

And that's exactly the way it went for the next year. Except for my regular visits to the Neurological Institute, I was able to put the whole matter out of my head, so to speak, and resume my life. I finished the Pollock biography (although, in places, it's not hard to tell what was on my mind as I was writing. Consider the following description of the artist creating one of his famous "drip" paintings: "The lines rose and fell, twisted and coiled, dividing like arteries or ending abruptly in bursts of black. Where there had been delicate webs, he wound dense, taut, capillary tangles.") Steve and

I started another book while that one wended its way through the editing process.

Then, in late 1989, just about the time the Pollock book was released, we left New York and bought a big, dilapidated country house in, of all places, Aiken, South Carolina, a little town near the Georgia border. I convinced myself that the quiet and simplicity of country life would, in some woolly, Thoreauesque way, be good for my health, even though I would have to return to the city every six months to keep my "contract" with Dr. Hilal.

For another year, the scans set off no alarms; the tumor stayed quiet. It was still there, of course, still growing, but only in unthreatening directions. Still no ticking. Meanwhile, Steve and I did a publicity tour for Pollock, worked on renovating the South Carolina house, and started yet another book. There were times, even, when I forgot the bomb altogether.

In April of 1991, the Pollock book won the Pulitzer Prize for biography (I told people that if the brain tumor had any side effects, they must have been good ones). When we scheduled our trip to New York for the prize ceremony at Columbia in September, I arranged another visit to Dr. Hilal's underground lair only a few blocks away. I had the scans taken before the ceremony but didn't have time to wait for the results, so I promised to come back afterward for the usual "where do we go from here" confab.

As soon as the ceremonies ended, I returned to the grotto with a signed copy of the book: "To Dr. Sadek Hilal, without whose help and concern and skill this book would not have been possible." He read the inscription without expression as he motioned me into his office. I was in such high spirits that I didn't register the grave look on his face until the moment he said the words that went with it: "I'm afraid I have bad news."

The bomb had started ticking.

ELEVEN

To Be, or Not to Be?

THIS TIME, I knew exactly what to do. No panic, no cinnamon buns, no lonely hotel rooms, no desperate phone calls home. Steve and I were prepared. We had foreseen this day and had the options ready: radiation, implantation, radiosurgery, old-fashioned surgery (heroic or otherwise), and, of course, nothing.

Now all I had to do was choose between them.

But how? How *is* one supposed to make these life-and-death decisions?

It's a question faced by every patient with a serious illness, but for which there is virtually no guidance out there: No "model" for decision making, as lawyers would say; no "decision tree," as businessmen would say. I know. I looked. A lot of patients, like me, are used to making their own decisions — financial, personal, professional, whatever — everything from "Should I start looking for another job?" to "What kind of car should I buy?" But medical decisions are something else entirely. Not only are the consequences so much more dire, but good information — the foundation of any good decision — is so much harder to come by. A person can follow the ups and downs of the job market or read *Consumer Reports*, but how does one know for sure if this surgical procedure will result in neurological damage or that kind of radiation will shrink a tumor and by how much?

Dr. James Kirklin, the heart surgeon, is only one of the more prominent voices in a chorus of lamentation over the lack of what is known in medical circles as "outcomes research." "You would be amazed," says Kirklin, "that for many, many kinds of surgical or medical options, such data have never been generated. You would think it would be automatic. You would think you ought to be able to punch into a computer your patient's characteristics and have the computer generate a profile based on multivariable analysis that would give you the expected outcomes with each given therapeutic option."

Imagine.

I walk to my local library and, using their computer, tap into an "Outcomes Data Bank" at the NIH. The screen displays a series of questions relating to "patient characteristics" (age, sex, weight, occupation, etc.), then instructs me to enter "nature of affliction/ illness/disease." When I type "brain tumor," another series of questions appears: type of tumor, level of aggressiveness, size, location, previous history and treatment, symptoms, etc. Finally, the screen prompts me to "Enter therapeutic option."

I type "conventional radiation," and the following screen appears:

Expected Outcomes: Conventional Radiation

Cure Rates (Reduction in Tumor Size)

total (100%)	6%
substantial (70 – 99%)	15%
partial (40 – 69%)	24%
some (20 – 39%)	22%
slight (1–19%)	28%
no effect (0%)	5%

Survival Rates

procedure	99%
hospital	98%
one-year	78%
two-year	41%
five-year	35%

For further information, click "Complications"

When I click "Complications," the screen lists them in order of likelihood, along with the percentage of patients who experienced them: eyesight impairment (22 percent), facial paralysis (35 percent), stroke (15 percent), memory loss (29 percent), and "other neurological damage" (37 percent). I request a hard copy of that information to read over more carefully at home, then move on to the next therapeutic option: surgery.

The screen displays another set of probabilities:

Expected Outcomes: Heroic Surgery

Cure Rates (Reduction in Tumor Size)

total (100%)	30%
substantial (70 – 99%)	36%
partial (40 – 69%)	26%
some (20 – 39%)	8%
slight (1–19%)	0%
no effect (0%)	0%

Survival Rates

procedure	85%
hospital	75%
one-year	33%
two-year	32%
five-year	29%

What does all this tell me? The chances of a complete cure are better with surgery, but so are the chances of dying in the hospital. Radiation has marginally better long-term survival figures

(35 percent were alive at the five-year mark, as opposed to 29 percent for surgery), but if I have the surgery and make it past the one-year mark, I will be more or less home free (only four out of thirty-five surgery patients, or roughly 10 percent, died between year one and year five, while more than 50 percent of radiation patients died in the same period).

And what about complications? The statistics tell me that 76 percent of the surgery patients experienced some kind of serious neurological damage, while only 32 percent of the radiation patients did. Furthermore, almost half (47 percent) of the surgery patients reported "memory loss or other cognitive problems," as opposed to only 17 percent of the radiation patients. That clinches it for me. I have my answer. I call Dr. Hilal and give him my decision.

Someday, maybe; but not yet.

I only *wish* I had had statistics like that when I was trying to decide what to do next. Who wouldn't want to have that kind of hard data when making a decision as important as how to deal with a brain tumor? But until the day Dr. Kirklin's fantasy becomes a reality, the question remains: How *should* a patient faced with a life-threatening illness go about choosing between various options for treatment?

Dr. Kirklin recommends starting with whatever information *is* available. "I see patients all the time who have been told only that they have 'a heart problem,' and given some medications, and that's it," says Kirklin. "No one has ever sat them down and told them, 'The natural history of your disease is the following, with and without treatment, and here are the things that could happen to you. Here's the probability of your living just one year. This is how many patients like you have survived for ten years with just standard therapy. These are your other therapeutic options. These are the expected outcomes or the possible outcomes with each.'

That's the kind of thing that every doctor should do, but they don't."

Or they can't.

There is one area of medicine, however, where that kind of information is available; where Dr. Kirklin's fantasy of decision making is almost a reality: transplants.

In 1978, Ann Harrison was diagnosed with alpha 1-antitrypsin deficiency, a rare lung disease even more devastating than emphysema. The doctors told her she had "the lungs of a seventy-five-year-old woman." She was thirty-three. "They told me there was nothing they could do for me," Harrison recalls, "and that I would never see my fiftieth birthday. I went home and I cried and cried and cried."

Then she heard about a doctor who just happened to be in the Harrisons' hometown, Toronto, who was looking for volunteer patients for a brand-new, untested procedure: double lung transplants. The doctor was Joel Cooper. At first, Harrison didn't take it seriously. New lungs? How could they possibly remove both her lungs and keep her alive while they inserted and connected another pair? And that was before she heard that the operation also included a piece of the donor's *heart!* It sounded, at best, daring; at worst, foolhardy.

Cooper didn't disagree. He told Harrison right out that there was only a "two percent chance of survival," Harrison remembers. "After all, I was the first double, and they had only done a very few singles before."

But what were the alternatives? By the time she found Dr. Cooper, Harrison had almost forgotten what it felt like to take a good deep breath. She was on oxygen twenty-four hours a day. A trip across the room was a struggle; a flight of stairs, unthinkable. She couldn't be left alone. "It gets to the point where people are doing everything for you," she recalls, "helping you get dressed, helping you wash. It's so degrading." When her husband, a teacher, wasn't home, her oldest son had to stay with her. When his high school friends called and asked him to go out, he would tell them, "No, I can't. You have to come over here." When she did go out, even to the store, she had to take her oxygen tank with her. "I'd be standing in line waiting to pay," she recalls, "and people would be so intimidated by the oxygen, nobody would ever talk to me."

Hardly a day passed without some kind of respiratory emergency. Not all of them required trips to the hospital, but many did, and every time she was rushed off to the emergency room gasping for breath, her ten-year-old retarded son thought she would never come back. At one of the pretransplant screenings with her family, a psychiatrist asked her if they had talked about the possibility of her dying and made funeral arrangements. Her retarded son jumped up and ran from the room. When Harrison's husband caught up to him in the hall, he just kept repeating, "I'm not going to talk about it. I'm not going to talk about it!"

Compared to that, even the prospect of not seeing her fiftieth birthday began to look attractive. "I just wanted to die," Harrison recalls. Until they told her *how* she would die. "They told me that when I went, I was going to go by suffocation. That's the way people with my problem die. They were very graphic about explaining that this was the way I was going to die if I didn't have this operation done."

For Harrison, the decision was easy, even without benefit of statistics or computers. "I don't want to live the way I'm living," she told Dr. Cooper. "I'd rather take my chances on the table. A two percent chance at something better is a whole lot better than a hundred percent chance at nothing, which is what I have now."

Ann Harrison beat the odds and, more than a decade after her double lung transplant, is alive to tell about it. In that decade, though, the transplants performed by Dr. Cooper and others have produced an extraordinarily detailed record that comes as close as anything in medicine to Dr. Kirklin's ideal of outcomes research databanks to help patients make informed decisions. "Because transplants are such a new procedure," says Cooper, "we have the best figures in the world. Of the last 250 transplants we've done, ninety-four percent have gone home after the operation. So there's only six percent mortality."

Also consistent with Dr. Kirklin's fantasy, experience has given doctors like Cooper (and, by extension, their patients) a more precise and predictable understanding of the complications arising from transplants. Indeed, so precise and predictable that those complications are themselves now commonly referred to as "transplant disease." "The transplant is a disease as well as the treatment," says Cooper, "because it's a new condition which has its own problems: a battery of medicines, some of them with possible complications; regular medical supervision for the rest of your life; and the ever-present danger of rejection."

Where Ann Harrison made a leap into the dark, transplant patients today make an enlightened trade-off: one disease for another; emphysema for transplant disease; cystic fibrosis for transplant disease; alpha 1-antitrypsin deficiency for transplant disease. They are informed up front of the procedure's risks and survival rates as well as the drawbacks of a "degraded lifestyle" afterward — like drug dependency. Ann Harrison suffers from osteoporosis in her feet and knees, and has had surgery for cataracts, all because of the steroids she takes. "But," says Harrison firmly, "it's a trade-off. I'd rather have sore feet and be a little bit shortsighted and be alive."

In fact, *every* decision about medical care involves "trade-offs." Whether it's trading one disease for another, or, as in my case, trading present or threatened ailments for future complications. Where the present ailment is intolerable (as in Ann Harrison's case) or the threatened one unacceptable (as in my case, before the first embolization), the decision is relatively easy: Almost any option is an attractive option. As Harrison puts it, "The fact that there was a possible solution overwhelmed the fear and the anxiety about the procedure. I just kind of sat there thinking, well, I'm going to die if I don't have something done, so why not." Joan Teckman, the swimmer who was diagnosed with cystic fibrosis, had a sister who died of CF. Her decision to have a lung transplant wasn't hard. "I just hoped and prayed that I was going to be accepted in the program," she told me. "I mean, that's all I wanted, because I knew that this was my only option for any kind of real life."

That feeling, that *certainty,* is typical of transplant patients. "I don't think there is a lung transplant patient anywhere," says Ann Harrison, "who could ever say that they had to think twice about doing it. Every one of them says, 'When can I have it? Yesterday?'"

But transplants are the exception. They're the easiest case, both because the trade-off is so dramatic, and because good information is so readily available. Much more typical is the decision I faced: What to do about a tumor that was growing in dangerous but unpredictable directions.

On the one hand, unlike Ann Harrison, I wasn't suffering. Indeed, my life was just getting back to normal. Yet all the treatment options available to me involved the risk of serious complications (paralysis, blindness, memory loss), complications that would cause suffering and could "degrade" my lifestyle in a massive way. What kind of trade-off was that? On the other hand, this tumor had a history of surprising me if I ignored it for too long. If I waited for the first sign of neurological problems before undergoing treatment, it might be too late. As if to remind me of that, I began experiencing brief spells of disorientation — like mild marijuana highs — soon after the post-Pulitzer meeting with Dr. Hilal. He suspected these "seizures," as he called them, were the first sign of the tumor's opening forays into the areas of my brain that controlled perception.

On the *other* hand, none of the treatment options I was considering held out much promise of a permanent solution. Nobody was claiming that radiation, radiosurgery, implantation, or even heroic surgery could *rid* me of this tumor; indeed, after my experience with the surgeon at U.C.L.A., I would have been suspicious if they had made such claims. Instead, Hilal and others talked about "retarding" the tumor's growth, or "shrinking it" or "reducing it" or, my personal favorite, "debulking it." I could see running the risk of massive neurological damage in pursuit of a permanent solution. The prospect of a life, even a degraded one, without this sword of Damocles hanging over me was mightily attractive: to rest assured that I would never have to do battle with this tumor again; to go to bed at night and not have to worry about whether my face, my eyes, my brain would work in the morning. *That* was a future worth taking risks for, even big risks. But for just another few years? Whatever happened, I didn't want to find myself five years later in exactly the same predicament, facing exactly the same decision, with exactly the same options — only no longer able to speak or see or remember anything that had happened in those five years.

What a mess. As decisions go, it was about as far from Dr. Kirklin's fantasy of rational, informed decision making as one could get. Instead of a neat printout of possible outcomes and complications with percentages for each that could be weighed and compared, I was looking at a page filled with *blanks:* variables, unknowns, unknowables, and imponderables. Next to this, my decision to do the first experimental embolization with Dr. Hilal looked like a lead-pipe cinch. There, the danger was clear, the risks acceptable, the options minimal, the procedure viable, and the benefits substantial. Here, every question led to a blank, it seemed, or just another question; and every effort to think it through sank in a morass of maybes, what ifs, but thens, and on the other hands. Like a lot of patients, I felt like I was trying to make a decision in a void.

But I *had* to make a decision.

So I did the only thing I could do: I tried to fill in as many of those blanks as possible.

I started by revisiting my options. In the five years since my Christmas trip to Mayo, I had learned a lot about the medical profession. Some people make a career out of their illnesses. I made a book. Not out of my illness, actually, more out of my search for doctors to treat my illness. After nine years and four editions of *The Best Lawyers in America,* Steve and I had begun work on the obvious companion volume, *The Best Doctors in America.* Beginning with the lists we had gathered in desperation at the kitchen table during my last medical crisis — the lists that led to Dr. Hilal — we spent two years subjecting the medical profession to the same nationwide polling process that we had perfected over the years with lawyers. In an effort to be comprehensive (the first edition included 3,200 doctors in 350 specialties), of course we learned much that wasn't relevant to my case. But the most important lesson we learned was: Never stop looking. And if you can't find what you need, wait a decade (if you can), or even just a few years. Medicine changes faster than fashion. A decade is a lifetime in medical-technology years — and can often make the difference between life and death.

Even in just the five years since I had first canvassed the country in search of treatment options, much had changed. Radiation techniques had evolved to new levels of subtlety and sophistication. The technology for shaping "fields" of radiation to conform to the shape of irregular tumors like mine, thereby minimizing the damage to sensitive surrounding tissue, had vastly improved. The once "radical" idea of implanting radioactive "seeds" had become an established, if not yet standard, technique for treating deep-brain tumors, and radiosurgery, that Scandinavian import, had attracted devotees and even whole departments in a number of medical centers around the country. It had, indeed, gone mainstream.

But nothing had changed more than neurosurgery. In only five years, tremendous advances in surgical techniques had made it possible for surgeons to operate in parts of the brain that had been off-limits only five years before, rendering some once "inoperable" brain tumors, miraculously, "operable."

Was mine one of them?

Using the list of neurosurgeons we had developed for *Best Doctors,* I found Dr. Vinko Dolenc, a native of Slovenia (formerly a part of Yugoslavia), and the undisputed expert at removing tumors in and around the area of the brain called the cavernous sinus. In fact, my tumor sprawled over a lot of area, but the only place it posed a real threat — the threat that had caused Dr. Hilal to sound the alarm — was in this tiny area with the improbable name. Through dissections on hundreds of cadavers — and a number of live patients as well (encouragingly, almost all of the latter had survived), Dr. Dolenc had developed a procedure for gaining access to this inaccessible area — thus making the inoperable operable. Even Dr. Hilal, who originally wanted me to have the surgery done at Columbia-Presbyterian, had to agree that Dolenc was "the number one guy."

This wasn't "heroic" surgery, either, at least not in the sense I had come to understand it. Dolenc wasn't interested in taking the top of my head off, scraping out the inside of my skull like a bowl of icing, then reattaching it — damn the neurological consequences — just to prove it could be done. What Dolenc did was the finest, most precise kind of microsurgery, based not on guts (the patient's) or glory (the doctor's), but on the finesse of an artist, the hands of a watchmaker, and an extraordinarily subtle and sensitive understanding of the microanatomy of this tiny, elusive junction box of nerves and blood vessels with the big-sounding name.

Dolenc was definitely a surgeon for the jet age. Although formally affiliated with the University of Virginia in this country, he performed surgery like an international rock star, traveling from hospital to hospital — Tel Aviv, Budapest, Vienna, Zurich, Stockholm, Paris, London, Milan, Madrid, Buenos Aires, Rio de Janeiro, São Paulo, Seoul, Tokyo, as well as his native Ljubljana — dazzling the local neurosurgeons at every stop with his impeccable technique, his encyclopedic knowledge, his remarkable stamina (six, seven, eight hours at a stretch), and his amazing results. With such global demand for his services, Dolenc had, in just a few years, performed more operations in the cavernous sinus than all the other surgeons in the world combined. He had even written a book about it called, aptly enough, *The Cavernous Sinus*. And when that became a bestseller, followed it up with a sequel, *Anatomy and Surgery of the Cavernous Sinus*.

This was, indeed, the guy who "wrote the book."

Only a few days after I sent my scans to him in Virginia, he called. "Yes," he said in a thick, Transylvanian accent (I imagined Bela Lugosi in white lab coat). "I can do this surgery."

Now the only question was: Did I *want* to do this surgery?

TWELVE

Balancing Act

SOONER OR LATER, the moment of decision comes: the moment when every option has been developed, every protocol and procedure researched, the best doctors chosen, all the available statistics gathered, and every blank that can be filled, filled. Sooner or later, every patient has to make the kind of calculation I did. What are the possible benefits of this treatment (procedure, protocol, whatever)? What are the likely costs? Can I live with those costs? Just how "possible" are those benefits and how "likely" are those costs? And then do the same for every option (for me, radiation, implantation, radiosurgery, neurosurgery, and, of course, doing nothing).

In the end, it's a balancing act.

And a delicate one. Too often, patients eager to arrive at one conclusion or another overvalue benefits and minimize costs — or vice versa. They "juggle the books," as one doctor put it. The sensitive scales of decision making can be upset by something as selfish as vanity ("I don't want to lose my hair!"), or as selfless as the convenience of family and friends ("I don't want them to have to travel to visit me").

I spoke to one patient who had suffered a cerebral hemorrhage and was deciding whether or not to have major surgery to correct the arterial defect in his brain that had caused it. The potential benefits of the procedure were overwhelming (e.g., survival), while the risks of serious complications were minimal. His surgeon estimated the chance of a "catastrophic outcome" at "around two percent"—remarkably good odds for major brain surgery. But the patient still balked. Why? He was worried about *his left foot.*

It seemed that the location of the defect would require the surgeon to retract the part of the brain that controlled motor function in the left foot. The patient was a twenty-two-year-old college student with an active lifestyle: hiking, skiing, playing tennis, lifting weights. "I was extremely worried about my left foot," he told me. "I wanted to do sports. I was active." The doctor tried to explain that, even if there was some damage, he would almost certainly still be able to walk without a detectable limp, he just might not have the fine coordination he was used to. But the prospect of not being able to schuss down the advanced slopes or do squat lifts with three hundred pounds was enough to paralyze this patient's decision-making process.

Compare that to another patient I spoke to, an elderly woman, who, when told that the course of chemotherapy she was considering would probably cause her hair to fall out, expressed shock that such a minor consequence would even be mentioned: "Who cares about my hair," she snapped. "I want to see my grandchildren!"

For many patients, though, myself included, vanity issues are the hardest. Even people who don't think of themselves as vain can discover deep reservoirs of vanity (fed, typically, by streams of insecurity) when threatened with the body-altering consequences of medical treatment. Whether it's something temporary, like hair loss, or permanent, like disfigurement; whether it's minor, like a visible scar, or major, like a missing breast; a limp or a limb, it matters. Regardless of how much the doctor or family and friends dismiss it as "purely cosmetic," it matters. If something *inside* is

156

altered (a missing kidney, a mechanical valve, a breast implant, another person's heart), that's okay, that's bearable. As long as it's not visible. Even pain, as bad as it is, is still a private burden. But something that can be seen by everyone who passes you on the street, something that permanently alters the way other people perceive you, *that* can carry more weight in the decision-making process than anything else — far more than it should.

For me, it was paralysis. When I surveyed the whole range of possible "complications" that might result from any of the treatments I was contemplating, the one that always sent a shudder of dread through me was facial paralysis. Partly, I think, because I had already been through it, if only for a while, and knew what a devastating effect it could have. Not a physical effect. Nothing that would bring me even one day closer to death. Indeed, it posed no real threat to my health at all, as long as I taped my eye shut every night. But what it did to my self-esteem — my sense of self — was truly murderous.

I would scold myself for the double standard I used in considering my afflictions — whether recalling past ones, bemoaning current ones, or weighing future ones. I had lived for years with a progressive bone disease that, if unchecked, *could* kill me, but I hardly ever thought about that. One of my ears was totally useless — but as long as nobody noticed . . . I knew it was shallow of me to care so much about "cosmetic" ailments, but I couldn't help it. I was haunted by visions of myself as a grotesque old hermit, living in a remote house with the windows heavily curtained, the lights turned low, and the mirrors all covered up, one side of my face withered with disuse, a patch over my dried-up eyeball, talking out of one side of my mouth, frightening to small children, disgusting even to friends, and turning into a person who existed solely on the telephone — only I couldn't talk on the telephone, either, because I couldn't talk.

This was my greatest fear: the fear that I fought to keep out of my decision-making process. But every time I tried to think through my options and decide on a treatment, it would rise darkly in the midst of my elegant ratiocinations and send all my carefully balanced, well-informed thoughts scurrying for cover.

My imagination may be overactive, but it's hardly unique. Strange as it seems, it is common for patients with life-threatening illnesses to scare themselves to death, so to speak, with morbid visions of the future. Like the patient who, when she discovered she had breast cancer, immediately went out and bought a burial plot. "I find that one thing most intelligent people unfortunately tend to do," says Dr. Robert Brumback, the trauma surgeon at the University of Maryland, "instead of creating a spectrum of possible outcomes, which is what they should do, they will assume the worst-case scenario. I know I do. I think it makes us feel better when the worst-case scenario doesn't come around."

Perhaps. But in the meantime, the tendency to overreact or panic or fix on the bleakest scenarios in the face of a medical crisis can seriously distort the decision-making process. I know that if I had tried to choose a treatment while in the grip of one of my paranoid fantasies of disfigurement, it would have been an equally misshapen choice. "The first thing a patient has to do," says Dr. Dorothy White, the pulmonologist at Sloan-Kettering, "is try to deal with the facts as we know them, as opposed to assumptions. Unfortunately, when people are told they have cancer, for example, there is a tendency to basically despair and to make all sorts of decisions on the basis of that despair: 'I'm going to do nothing,' or 'This is hopeless,' or 'I'm not willing to do this, I'm not willing to take anything that makes me lose my hair, I'm not willing to do that.' Patients need to weigh the options, do some research, take stock, get the facts, and get past the panic, before making any decisions."

Catherine LeDuc knows what "the panic" feels like. She was twenty-eight, married only four years, and eager to start a family when she was diagnosed with "stage II adenocarcinoma of the cervix" — cervical cancer. First came the shock, then the revulsion, *then* the panic. "When I heard the bad news for the first time," she recalls, "I just wanted to find a solution, any solution, right away." Unfortunately, her doctors weren't much help. Even after a conization (a surgical procedure in which a sample of tumor is removed for testing), they couldn't tell her if the cancer was malignant or not. It might be, they waffled, but they couldn't be sure. She had three options, they said: She could do another conization, which might yield a more definitive answer to the question of malignancy; she could assume the cancer was malignant and go forward with a radical hysterectomy; or, of course, she could wait and do nothing.

"I don't feel I have the tools to make a decision," she told them.

"Well, it's up to you," they said.

Fighting her "natural instinct to panic," LeDuc sat down at her kitchen table with a piece of paper and made three columns. At the top of each column, she wrote one of her three options — "2nd Conization," "Hysterectomy," "Do nothing" — then listed the pros and cons of each. She tackled the easy one first: "Do Nothing — Pros." "No operation," she wrote, then "maybe get one child under the wire." But she didn't want to fool herself, so she added, "No guarantees," and then, after another long moment of reflection, "without mother?" Under "Do Nothing — Cons," she first wrote, "uncertainty," then crossed it out and wrote, "death," then added, "sooner or later."

Under "2nd Conization — Pros," she wrote, "Smaller surgery," and "Can still have children." Then she realized that if the cancer proved malignant and she had the hysterectomy, both those "pros" would be canceled out, so she wrote a big question mark in the margin beside them. Under "2nd Conization — Cons," she wrote, "gives the cancer more time to spread if malignant"; "also if malignant, have to do two operations instead of one, have hysterectomy anyway"; and, finally, "will have to wait even longer to find out about malignancy." Then, under the heading

"Hysterectomy — Pros," she wrote, "deal with cancer definitively, sooner," and "no more worry," and "gets it out" with an exclamation point. Under "Hysterectomy — Cons," she wrote just two words, and underlined them heavily, "No children."

Difficult as it was, Catherine LeDuc was only doing what doctors advise every patient to do. "The patient needs to put things into context," says Dr. Andrew von Eschenbach, the urologic surgeon, "and the context is the trade-off between what's to be gained and what price has to be paid, and it's always the patient who has to make the final determination." *What's to be gained versus what price has to be paid*. Benefits and costs. Von Eschenbach suggests to his patients that they think of the relationship between these two as a ratio. An option that has a high cost/benefit ratio would either be foolish not to do (when the benefits are great and the costs minimal) or foolhardy to do (when the benefits are minimal and the costs great).

Von Eschenbach uses as an example the disease he deals with every day, prostate cancer. "Whether a patient chooses to have surgery or do hormone therapy should depend on how advanced the cancer is," he explains. "There's no place for radical surgery in the presence of widespread metastasis because attacking a primary tumor when the cancer has already spread subjects the patient to all of the risks associated with the surgery and none of the benefits. So the ratio is very lopsided. The benefits as far as the outcome of the disease is concerned are nil and the risks are quite high. For hormone therapy, on the other hand, the ratio is very favorable. You can attack the cancer both in the prostate itself as well as at the distant metastatic sites, and you don't have any of the risks of surgery."

Of course, von Eschenbach adds, there are complications to consider. Hormone therapy produces "hot flashes," similar to those women experience during menopause, and there is some decline in sexual drive (although not, as many patients mistakenly believe, to the point of preventing normal sexual functions like erection, climax, and orgasm), and these may affect the "ratio" between costs and benefits. *How much* they affect it, however, depends on the patient. When faced with a choice between radiation therapy or radical surgery, some patients make their decision "purely on their perception of the side effects and how troublesome those side effects may be to them," says von Eschenbach.

The one especially "troublesome" side effect of prostate surgery that tips the balance for many patients is urinary incontinence. "They'll say, 'No, I absolutely don't want a radical prostatectomy if there's any chance of incontinence,'" according to von Eschenbach. "For them, that throws the ratio way out of balance. The possible benefits of surgery, no matter how great, are overwhelmed by the possible cost of incontinence. For some, that's just too high a price to pay." Von Eschenbach says he doesn't always agree with the balance his patients strike between costs and benefits, but he always leaves the final decision up to them. "As a physician," he says, "it's my responsibility to present the correct options with all the pluses and minuses and then let the patient determine what weight to assign them — how to calculate the ratio."

Von Eschenbach also notes that for some problems, especially chronic ones like mine, the ratio of costs to benefits can change over time. "Early in the illness there may be much to be gained and very little price to be paid for a particular treatment," he says. "But as the disease becomes more advanced and other treatments are used up or are no longer effective, the ratio changes. The possible benefits may get less possible and the likely costs may get more likely. There may be less assurance that the treatment will help, and more assurance that the side effects will be serious." For example, in my case, I knew that the longer I waited to do anything, the longer I gave the tumor to grow, the less effective conventional radiation would be. I also knew that if I waited until the tumor encroached on some nerve (like the optic nerve) or some sensitive area of the brain (like the cavernous sinus), then the possiblity of serious complications, especially neurological damage, from surgery would shoot up, because to get the tumor *out* of those areas, a surgeon would have to go *into* those areas.

The ratio can also change over time as patients become "fed up" with the price they have to pay in terms of discomfort or sacrifice to receive the benefits of certain treatments. "They decide enough's enough," says von Eschenbach. "They tell me, 'I'm not going to endure all the pain and all the suffering and all the costs that are associated with that treatment when I've already been though so much and the disease is so extensive and the likelihood of that particular treatment having a major benefit for me just doesn't seem to make it worthwhile anymore." So a favorable ratio becomes an unfavorable ratio.

Although I didn't know it at the time, that is more or less the way I thought about costs and benefits — on those rare occasions when I could beat back my fears and think rationally — as I contemplated my options after "the bomb" started ticking again. Would I accept a 40 percent risk of paralysis with a 60 percent chance of total cure? It was easy to set the boundaries. A 10 percent risk of serious damage and a 90 percent chance of cure? Easy. A 90 percent risk of damage with only a 10 percent chance of cure? Also easy. But what about 40/60 (40 percent risk of damage, 60 percent chance of cure)? Or 60/40? Where was the line? 30/70? What about 30/30? That was easy, too (no), but what about 30/50? And how did the answer change if the benefit side of the ratio wasn't total cure, but only partial cure? For instance, how about a 50 percent risk of damage for an 80 percent *reduction*? (Answer: no; that would only buy me time. Why take a big risk for just a few years?) And what if the cost side of the ratio wasn't total paralysis, but only partial paralysis? Or partial blindness?

Of course, the numbers I was working with were purely hypothetical. It was really more a mental exercise to get me thinking in terms of probabilities and trade-offs. But many of the doctors I spoke to agreed that patients have the right to demand not just generalities, but *percentages:* especially for the likelihood of a favorable outcome and for the chances of a serious complication. There's a catch, though. "If you have confidence in your doctor," says Dr. John Marini, director of pulmonary and critical care medicine at St. Paul–Ramsey Medical Center in Minnesota, "then you will allow that physician enough latitude to make intelligent guesses *and to be wrong about them.*" In other words, patients can press their doctors to guesstimate percentages as an aid in their decision making, but they need to understand that "guesses are guesses, not guarantees."

The other thing to remember is that, except in the easiest cases, there are no "right" answers. Because everybody suffers differently, everybody feels pain differently, everybody *fears* pain differently; because everybody fears different things, believes different things, hopes for different things, and can bear different things, *everybody's "balance" will be different.* Everybody will weigh probabilities differently, will calculate ratios differently, and will draw the line between what's acceptable and what's unacceptable at different places. "My experience," says Dr. W. Marston Linehan, the head of urologic oncology at NIH, "has been not so much that patients make the right decision. Sometimes, you know, only God knows the right decision. But sometimes they will make what *to them* is the right decision. And that's the important thing."

Some patients are natural risk-takers; some, risk-averse. Some patients are aiming for permanent cures, some for long remissions, some for just a few more years. Dr. Dorothy White notes that "younger patients tend to accept more rigorous therapies." I talked to a young patient who undertook an extremely rigorous and risky experimental multiple transplant because "the fact that I was contributing to something larger than myself gave me additional strength." But another patient might not give a fig about the advancement of medical science. "Patients have a tremendous need to express their wishes," says Dr. White, "and they should. Some will say, 'I want a chance to live, and I'm really willing to roll the dice to have even a small chance.' Others will say, 'I just don't want to go through a lot of things that may be of no benefit to me,' or, 'I really don't want to give up my hair now,' or, 'I don't want to take the risk that I will have complications down the line for something that's very uncertain now.' Everyone has to strike their own balance."

When Catherine LeDuc was trying to strike her balance, she was put in touch with another young woman who had recently faced the same decision. Like LeDuc, she had been married only a short time when she was diagnosed with cervical cancer. She, too, didn't know if her cancer was malignant when she had to make a decision. Her choice: hysterectomy. The woman told LeDuc that she was glad she chose to have the operation because, *for her,* the worst prospect was having to wait to find out if her cancer was malignant. "Talking to her helped me a lot," LeDuc recalls, "but her solution was too radical for me. If she had waited, who knows? But she didn't want to wait. Some people think about things differently than others." For LeDuc, waiting wasn't a problem — not nearly as much of a problem as "<u>No children.</u>" She chose to have the second conization and the resulting test showed that her cancer was not malignant. She never had a hysterectomy.

Transplant pioneer Ann Harrison tells the story of another transplant patient, also in her early thirties, who had the same disease as Harrison and was a candidate for the same procedure at about the same time. The only real difference was that this woman's children, at five and eight, were younger than Harrison's. "She had no problem with the transplant," Harrison recalls. "The hardest thing for her was being away from her kids back in Illinois for the months she had to wait for a donor. 'If I don't make it,' she said, 'then I've wasted those five or six months when I could have been with them.'" Still, she decided to go ahead and have the transplant with the help of strangers who dropped coins into special jars beside cash registers in stores throughout Illinois.

Today, the two women talk on the phone often. "Our phone bills are astronomical," says Harrison.

Harold Taylor, the wizard of London's Wall Street, brought his usual care and clear-headedness to the often murky business of balancing costs and benefits. "After understanding the disease to the best of your ability," he told me, "you have to recognize psychologically that there are no right answers. Even if I had been a myeloma specialist *myself,* it still wouldn't have been possible to say, 'Well, this is what I should do.'" So, like Catherine LeDuc, Taylor set out his three options on a piece of paper: "Conventional Chemotherapy," "Radiation," and "Radical Chemotherapy."

"Historically, conventional chemotherapy treatment of melphalan and prednisone have proved to have a very marked but short-term effect," Taylor explains. "Over the last twenty years, it has shown very little likelihood of producing a longer-term success. So we eliminated that because we weren't interested in just trying to buy two or three years of relief. We were looking for something altogether more effective, more in the nature of a home run."

The next option was radiation. "The problem with radiation," Taylor recalls, "is that by and large, once you have had it, that's it. You have used up that option. There is no going back on it. Unlike surgery or chemotherapy, that arrow is permanently gone from your quiver once you've shot it. So it seemed best to hold that back."

That left radical chemotherapy. "On the negative side," says Taylor, "experimental chemotherapy is more painful. But I asked myself, what kind of pain? Actually, it's more nauseating than painful. It's lassitude, it's depression, it's physical weariness and the loss of any sense of energy. But there are drugs that can mediate those effects." And on the positive side? "Radical chemotherapy, if administered at a place where they have experience in handling this sort of extreme regimen — you're not playing with aspirin here — at least held out the promise of a home run."

So what did he decide? How did he strike the balance? "In the end, we chose to go down the radical chemotherapy route and leave the radiation in reserve in case that should be needed later. That's what we chose to do."

For all three of these patients, Ann Harrison, Catherine LeDuc, and Harold Taylor, as for thousands of others like them, the act of choosing is, in itself, beneficial. "It is tremendously reassuring," says Taylor, "as you go through the subsequent treatment, to know that you have chosen as far as you are able the best thing to do, and that you have participated, you have been an active agent in getting to that position. It makes everything, from the waiting to the pain, much, much more bearable. If we had just sat here in the U.K. and said, well, the doctor recommends that we do this, or the doctor recommends we do that, and then just followed through, I don't think I would have felt nearly as brilliant or hopeful as I did."

And what about me? What did I do to make me feel "brilliant and hopeful"? Which way did the cost/benefit scales tip in my case?

I only wish I had possessed the conviction of Catherine LeDuc, the courage of Ann Harrison, or the conscientiousness of Harold Taylor. I never did pull out a piece of paper and make headings, or press my doctors to give me percentages for my calculations. But I did calculate. Like Ann Harrison, I calculated that the status quo *had* to change. Ever since the meeting with Hilal, the déjà vu–like spells had grown more frequent and more severe, and there were worrisome new signs of "trouble upstairs": sleeplessness, headaches, and facial "neuralgias" (a tingling like when your foot falls asleep). Clearly, I had to do something. Like Catherine LeDuc, I didn't want to panic and overreact — reach for a radical remedy, like heroic surgery, just because it held out the promise of "getting rid of this thing once and for all" — even if I believed that promise. And finally, like Harold Taylor, I thought I'd better hold something back for a rainy day. This tumor had proven a durable, persistent enemy over two decades, so I decided to keep radiation in reserve in case all else failed. (Besides, no one was making any promises for its effectiveness.)

After all that calculating, only one option was left standing: the globe-trotting Dr. Dolenc and his miraculous new procedure. It offered the potential for dramatic results without the dramatic risks of heroic surgery, the reliability of radiation without foreclosing later options, the robust promise of an innovative solution without the anemic record of radiosurgery or implantation. My conversations with Dr. Dolenc only reinforced the sense that I had discovered the trapdoor out of the room just as the fast-closing walls were about to crush me. Out of three hundred patients, operating in this incredibly sensitive, formerly "inoperable" part of the brain, Dolenc had lost only seven.

I set a date for the operation, then put the whole thing out of my head, so to speak, satisfied with my decision and confident that I had done my job well, and now it was over.

In fact, it had just begun.

THIRTEEN

The Right Stuff

A LOT OF patients, even conscientious, take-charge patients like Harold Taylor, even patients who doggedly follow every lead and research every possible treatment, even patients, like me, who enjoy partnerships with their doctors, have a tendency to think that once they make their decision about treatment, their job is over. After all that research and careful balancing of probabilities and agonizing trade-offs, they think they deserve a break. Finally, it's all in the doctor's hands. There's nothing more they can do.

Wrong.

All kinds of extravagant claims are being made these days for the importance of attitude: the power of positive thinking, the triumph of mind over body, etc., etc. And why not? There is no end of patients out there who claim that they willed their cancer into remission, or prayed their emphysema away, or visualized their tumor out of existence. "If your mind-set is that you're going to die, you're going to die," said one patient I spoke to, "and if your mind-set is that you're going to live, then you're going to live. It's as simple as that." He then recounted a story he had heard about a boy with cancer whose case "was considered hopeless." According to the story, this boy went to sleep one night saying, "I'm going to kill off all the bad cells in my body. I'm going to kill off all the bad cells in my body," repeating it over and over and over, "and he woke up the next morning without any cancer." Another patient told me about his father who, at age sixty, was diagnosed as "full of cancer" and given six months to live. *Without doing anything about it,* he lived another seveteen years, according to this story, and even then died of a non-cancer related illness. How? "He just made up his mind he was going to lick it."

Oh.

For a natural-born cynic like me, such stories always raised the hackles of skepticism. I thought they belonged on the front page of the *Enquirer* alongside the Elvis sightings and UFO babies. For a long time, in my world, there was no such thing as a medical miracle, only hard-won victories — and usually partial or temporary ones at that.

That kind of cynicism, however, is getting harder and harder to maintain, especially now that even doctors — reputable ones — are jumping on the "will yourself to wellness" bandwagon. "The psychological attitude of the patient is, believe it or not, the single most important determinant as to whether they get well or not," says Dr. Nicholas Gonzalez. "The brain is extraordinarily powerful. It can override what any doctor does biologically."

Of course, Dr. Gonzalez is a Manhattan-based expert in *alternative* medicine, so he might be expected to have fringe views on this issue, despite his rigorously orthodox research background. But *every* doctor I spoke to, from the most traditional to the most alternative, agreed with the basic sentiment: There is some kind of connection between the mind and the body, between attitude and healthy functioning, that, to varying degrees, affects the outcome of every case.

In a very unscientific way, doctors have known this for decades. Every doctor has stories of patients who, it seemed, *willed* themselves to survive, despite all the weight of medical facts against them. "I guess we're just beginning to come to grips with the observation," says Dr. Andrew von Eschenbach, the urologic surgeon. "But the phenomenon has been apparent for a long time to physicians who have had their eyes open, so to speak, and their minds open to these possibilities."

When pressed to go beyond anecdotal evidence, doctors like von Eschenbach usually talk in vague terms of immune response. "Clearly, there's some biologic process that allows a beneficial effect to take place," he says. "We realize that there's a connection between the brain and the nervous system and the immune system, that nerves interact with T cells, that sort of thing." Dr. Thomas Petty, the pulmonary expert at Presbyterian – St. Luke's in Denver, states the proposition more baldly. "Attitudinal change will alter your immune reactivity," says Petty. "Depressive people usually lose their immune responses and people who are on top of the world usually maintain their immune responses."

How does this mind-body immune system connection work? The closest thing to an explanation comes from Dr. W. Marston Linehan at NIH. "We know the immune system does surveillance in the body for cancer," says Linehan, "so it's not hard to understand how a patient with a depressed immune system, a patient who is very agitated or depressed, would not respond as well physically to his or her cancer as one who has a very positive frame of mind." Although, he adds, "I can't tell you how scientifically valid that observation is."

There's a lot of history in that caveat.

In fact, for all its current enthusiasm, mainstream medicine was slow to accept the psychological dimension of *illness* — much less cure. Dr. Samuel Klagsbrun, a psychiatrist at Four Winds Hospital in Katonah, New York, remembers when Memorial Sloan-Kettering, the huge cancer center in New York, had only one part-time psychiatrist on staff to treat patients — "and he was a rather depressed man himself." He also only worked half-time. "The bulk of the emotional and psychological work," Klagsbrun recalls, "was borne by a very sophisticated and unusually gifted group of social workers, who were themselves very depressed, by the way, because they were overwhelmed by the responsibilities thrust on them. The hospital was doing a lot of experimental stuff. The death rate was enormous. All the obvious things that created stress in that system were present."

The legacy of that initial skepticism can still be found in the medical community, just beneath the surface of open-mindedness. Largely because of the lack of scientific proof, there is still a good deal of ambivalence about the concept of "mind over matter" healing. One doctor referred to it as the "pornography" of medicine: "Physicians can't define it, but they know it when they see it." Listen to the ambivalence in the endorsement of Dr. Hermes Grillo, the eminent tracheal surgeon at Massachusetts General Hospital. "I think attitude makes a huge difference. Two weeks after an operation, one patient will be moaning and groaning and having a terrible time, while another patient will be asking me, 'Doc, is it all right if I go out and just play a few holes of golf?' There's no question. Positive attitude buoys people up and gets them through difficult times — although, frankly, I don't think it changes the outcome of the disease . . . well, we don't know that. We don't know what all the interrelationships are physiologically between attitudes and spirit and T-cell counts and whatnot."

Like Grillo, a lot of doctors tend to hedge their enthusiasm for this new branch of medicine with qualifiers and caveats. In addition to pleading the lack of hard evidence, they point out that the anecdotal patients are often self-selected. Or they concede the importance of attitude in the *recovery* process (from operations, for example), but not in the healing or curative process. It can "buoy people up and get them through difficult" ordeals, as Grillo says, but not necessarily alter the course of their disease. Others will attest from their own experience that patients can will themselves to *die*— that they can override medical advantages, medical help, even strenuous medical efforts in the opposite direction, and "cash out" — but are resolutely ambivalent on the other side of that coin: the patients' ability to hang on to life when all the medical facts are against them. "If a patient wants to die," says Dr. Gonzalez, "it's almost like voodoo, they're going to die no matter who treats them. I've had several patients who just really didn't want to live. They were just going through the motions, and no matter what you did the tumors got worse. It's amazing."

All this may sound like nothing more than professional turf-guarding — if patients can heal themselves with positive thoughts, where does that leave doctors? — but, in fact, I think many doctors see a real danger in making too much of this mind-body connection. "Unless you're very careful," one doctor told me, "patients end up getting blamed for their illness. You know, the simplistic approach that says cancer is the door of resentment, and all you have to do is get rid of that resentment and the cancer will go away. And if you don't, it won't." That is, after all, the logical extension of the "think yourself to health" argument. If positive thinking, or whatever, can make you well, then, if you don't get better, you must not be thinking positively enough. You must be doing something wrong. You don't really *want* to get well. And if you die, well, it's really your own fault.

"I think there is a very real sense in which determination and grit and a kind of fighting spirit help a person survive longer than the person who gives up and becomes despondent," says Dr. William Wood at Emory. "But I think that, if you carry that too far, then the patient feels guilty about being sick, and guiltiest of all when he's dying."

Dr. Madelon Baranoski, the former army nurse who served in Vietnam, believes strongly in the power of "a fighting spirit" — "What kept striking me over there was how effective the human will was," she recalls — but she deplores the implication that sickness represents a *failure* of spirit. "There's a kind of arrogance about it," she says, "blaming people for being sick. Telling them that, if you really had enough of that fighting spirit, you wouldn't be so sick. Some people get the message from these gurus that if you fail, then you're a failure. I think that's the wrong message. If you take a turn for the worse, it deprives you of your sense of hope because you now feel that you must have done something wrong. So you end up being a failure once again. And you're to blame for it."

Baranoski tells about a study done in Detroit and sponsored by the Big Three automakers to investigate why there was such a high incidence of colon cancer among autoworkers. Completely disregarding environmental factors like paint and noise and on-the-line stress, the study looked at the "personality structure" of the men who were suffering with colon cancer. "The whole study was designed to put across the companies' argument that all this environmental stuff had nothing to do with it," says Baranoski. "If these men got cancer, it was their own fault. It wasn't the companies' fault."

One patient I spoke to assailed the arrogance of people who take credit for having lived through a life-threatening illness, thereby putting blame on all those people who don't survive for having failed to live, comparing it to the arrogance of a relative of hers who won the lottery and "actually felt that he got credit for having won, that this somehow enhanced him as a person."

This same patient told me about a friend of hers — her "closest friend in the whole world," mentor, spiritual sister, and godmother of her children — who discovered she had a kidney tumor. She went to the best hospitals, got the best doctors, had all the best care, and, according to this woman, "had an incredible spirit and will to live. I've never seen anybody want to live more." She had five or six operations and died within eighteen months "in the most horrible way — not just physically horrible, but also morally horrible, because she was really sure she was going to be able to survive, and it didn't work. And I refuse to believe that it was her fault — in any way. She had all the fighting spirit in the world."

What does it mean to "have fighting spirit"?

The woman who told me that story knows.

Alice Trillin was thirty-eight and feeling great when she coughed up a tiny blood clot. More curious than concerned, she went to her regular internist, who did a routine chest x-ray that changed Trillin's life. "Lo and behold, there was this weird-looking thing in my lungs," she recalls. Even when she scheduled the surgery to have that weird-looking thing removed, she wasn't worried. "I certainly didn't think I had cancer," she says. "How could somebody have lung cancer at thirty-eight who had never smoked? Nobody thought I had cancer."

But she did. Malignant adenocarcinoma, to be specific, and it had spread to her lymph nodes. Her doctors put her through the usual wringer of radiation and chemotherapy — this was 1976, before they knew that chemotherapy was often ineffective against lung cancer — and when those didn't work, tried some experimental immunotherapy. "They were throwing everything they could at this disease," Trillin recalls, "because the prognosis wasn't great."

But Trillin was looking for more than just protocols for her cancer. As a writer (as well as the wife of a writer), she wanted protocols for her mind as well. "I kind of wanted a philosophy of cancer," she says, "as well as a medical approach. I felt it was important to know how to think about this." At first, her doctor wasn't much help. "He tried to make me feel like it was my fault that I had the disease," she recalls. "I asked him some questions, like what kind of protocols do you have, and he yelled at me, 'Well, if you think this is going to go away like the common cold, young lady, you've got another think coming.'"

Trillin wasn't about to take that from anyone, even a doctor. "I had a rule," she says. "When I got someplace I didn't like, I left."

She left that doctor in a hurry and, fortunately, ended up at Memorial Sloan-Kettering in the care of Dr. Mark Meyers, a very different kind of caregiver. "I saw this man, and it was like my life turned around," Trillin recalls. "He made me feel as if I had control over my own treatment, as if he would do everything within his power to help me." Finally, her spirit, as well as her body, was in good hands.

Not a minute too soon. Alice Trillin spent the next fifteen years in hell. Nothing seemed to work, and everything that could go wrong, every complication that could arise, did. Two years of additional chemotherapy left her blood so depleted that her doctors suspected her bone marrow wasn't functioning. They feared all the treatments had given her leukemia. A biopsy was negative, but the medication they gave her resulted in "instant menopause." Then one day she felt a spasm that began in her neck and ended up in her feet. She knew that one of the first places lung cancer goes is to the brain. "I just thought this was probably it," she recalls.

But it was another false alarm — "just" a degeneration of the nerves in the cervical spine caused by radiation. Then, only five years ago, after a bad case of pleural effusion (fluid on the lungs) she was told she had a recurrence. The cancer had not only returned but had metastasized to her bones — a not uncommon but often fatal twist in long-term cancer patients like Trillin. "That definitely should have been the end of my life," she says. The only solution, the doctors told her, was a thoracotomy, a major operation to remove the tumors altogether. And if that wasn't bad enough, one of the tumors was compressing her spinal cord in a way that might quickly lead to paralysis. Even if she survived the cancer, she might spend the rest of her life as a paraplegic.

Then, on the eve of surgery, the doctors decided they had made a mistake. Those were not tumors on her x-rays, those were fractures. The premature menopause had ushered in premature osteoporosis and her weakened bones had cracked during the violent coughing fits that accompanied her bout of pleural effusion. "Or at least that was their best guess," she says.

Defying all the odds and all her doctors' predictions, Alice Trillin is still alive, twenty years after her original diagnosis. So startling is her survival that doctors have periodically gone back to review her original x-rays "just to be sure that no mistake was made in diagnosing the disease," according to one of her doctors. There was no mistake. "Mrs. Trillin had lung cancer at a time when, even more than today, it was considered an instantly terminal disease," says the doctor, Dorothy White. "It had spread to her lymph nodes, which usually means an extremely poor prognosis. Most patients who have that will succumb to their disease. She is definitely a survivor. She got very good treatment and very aggressive treatment, but, in fairness, there are other people who got that and did not survive."

Why? What was Alice Trillin's secret? What did she have that those other patients didn't have? Trillin is suspicious of questions like that. "It's really not something that you can take credit for," she says. "I think that you can take credit for doing it well, either dying well or surviving with the best possible life. But there's a major element of luck. It's a little bit like a slot machine in Las Vegas, where, if all the oranges click into place at the same time, you get to go home, but if you've got one orange and a couple of bananas or something, then you die." *But,* Trillin adds, she believes it *is* possible to "shift the balance a little" to make it more likely that those three oranges will pop into place; in short, to improve the odds of winning the jackpot.

That's where the "compulsion to live" comes in.

Trillin's compulsion sprang from two sources. The first was her unshakable faith in the power of the mind. "I'm a great believer in rational approaches to solving problems," she says. "I have always lived by my head rather than my body. I'm a problem solver. And I believe that there are two kinds of problems: the ones that have no good answers — there's no way out of them — and all the others. You just take each problem one step at a time and if you're not happy with the way it is, you just have to try to change it."

Trillin thinks that perhaps her quasi-religious devotion to the power of rational problem solving is the flipped legacy of a childhood in which problems never got solved. "I grew up in a family where people were never totally in control," she recalls. "My parents were always floundering around." Her father lost all of his money and her mother never did anything to make her own life better. She even had trouble getting pregnant and giving birth. Years later, when Trillin started her own family, she thought, "What's the big deal? I got pregnant the first week I tried and had my baby in four hours of labor." While she concedes that it isn't possible "to control precisely the duration of one's labor psychologically," she remains convinced "that all those things that had been such a big deal to my parents had to be easier to control," and she still believes that there is very little in life that won't yield to a sustained, rational effort at solution.

The other source of Trillin's compulsion to live was more commonplace: her children. "I had this great life," she says. "I mean, I had this great husband, but mainly I had these great children. I can't say this, even now, without wanting to cry. But I could not leave them. I just could not leave them. Once you're a parent, you really do feel you have these messages to pass on, and you're not immortal if you don't get to pass them on to somebody. That was my real compulsion to live. I told my husband, 'If there's any kind of lifeline here, I will grab it.'"

Alice Trillin uses the term "compulsion to live." Other patients and other doctors use other terms, but they all come down to the same thing: the need to fight — physically, emotionally, psychologically. "We have a term here for patients who are fighters," says heart surgeon James Kirklin. "We say they 'come to play.' Some patients come to play and some just come to sit on the bench."

One fact is undeniable. In the battle against life-threatening illness, victory goes to those who "come to play." "There are just some patients who mobilize their resources," says Dr. Andrew von Eschenbach, the urologic surgeon, "and instead of the cancer attacking them, they start attacking the cancer. And those are often the ones left standing at the end of the day, totally free of disease, and, scientifically speaking, it's difficult to justify how."

Dr. Baranoski and a team of researchers at Yale did a study of melanoma patients, starting at the point of diagnosis and following them for several years afterward. They asked the attending physicians to make predictions about how well they thought their patients would do with this aggressive cancer *based solely on the patient's response* at the time of diagnosis. "We matched patients for type of tumor, level of invasion, treatment regimen, and so on," explains Baranoski, "so the doctors were just looking at the way the patients were responding to their illness, focusing on their psychology, and making an estimate about how well they were going to do."

Baranoski discovered not only that the doctors' predictions were usually wrong (heartening news to anybody who has been given three months to live by a grim-faced doctor), but also that "the people who were most upset at the time of the diagnosis, the ones who decided right up front that they weren't going to accept it, *those* were the ones who ended up having the best long-term outcomes." And who had the worst outcomes? "The people who said, well, okay, you know, so I have cancer. It's not going to bother me."

Baranoski remembers one woman in particular. "She just said, 'Well, okay, I'm just not going to think about it. It's not going to affect my life. It would just destroy my husband.' She was one of the people whose melanoma later metastasized and she died."

At first, Baranoski and her fellow researchers were startled by the results. They seemed "counterintuitive," she recalls. The accepted wisdom had always been that the poised, serene patient was more likely to bear the heavy and sometimes horrific burdens of both the disease and its treatment. The patient who wasted precious energy on anger and denial would quickly burn out. "But when we looked at it more closely," Baranoski remembers, "we thought, wait a minute. What are we talking about here? What does it mean to 'accept' your illness? Accepting your illness is sort of putting it aside and not dealing with it, the way a lot of people deal with stress. They just put it aside, until eventually it erupts as an illness or a psychological problem." In order to truly fight the illness, physically and emotionally, a patient "needs to be pretty angry about it," says Baranoski. Some of the patients who eventually had positive long-term outcomes didn't feel the anger right away. They went through an initial period of "disorganization," according to the study, a period characterized by "hopelessness and helplessness." But eventually they all came around to the anger that motivated them to what Baranoski calls "the struggle."

Their struggles took different forms. "Some people used information," says Baranoski. "They tried to find out everything they could about their disease. They had a sense that the cancer was something that could be defeated by gaining power over it, and information gave them that power. Others decided that they knew their own body, and so they would do whatever they needed to do to take control of their body back from the disease. For some, that meant changing diets; for others, relaxation therapy; for others, finding constructive outlets for their anger. But everybody was *doing* something to reassert control as a way of fighting the disease."

Does that mean that denial is a good thing?

Like a lot of patients, I had always thought of denial as something to be avoided. People who "lived in denial" were people who didn't face up to their problems, whether those problems were serious illness, antisocial habits, or self-destructive relationships. I had lived in denial for a long time before that fateful Christmas party. The gurus at Mayo were telling me what I wanted to hear — no recurrence of the tumor — which made it easy for me to ignore the continuing problems in my blood and bones. After the party, of course, the facial paralysis made denial impossible. But after the first embolization, as consonants reappeared in my speech and control returned to my smile, I could feel the denial creeping back in, too.

Even after Dr. Hilal sounded the second alarm, I looked and felt better than I had in years. I had been to the Pulitzer ceremony, read an excerpt from the Pollock biography to a crowd at the National Book Awards dinner, given a speech at my college, and *nobody noticed anything wrong.* Maybe there *wasn't* anything wrong. I never talked about my long medical ordeal. New friends were surprised when they found out about it ("You had *brain* surgery?"), which always gave me strange satisfaction. I never retreated so far into denial that I lied about it, but when I went to my twentieth high school reunion, *I never mentioned it.* I treated it like a test. (Audrey Hepburn in *My Fair Lady.* Would they notice?) But it was also a temptation, a temptation to forget yet again about that awful Christmas.

To me, that's what denial is: a kind of willful blindness, a forced forgetfulness. (And an irritable one, too. Woe to anyone who tries to bring the light of truth to a person living in the darkness of denial.) And if a patient refuses to see his problem, how can he begin to solve it? The better course, I always thought, was to calmly accept reality, no matter how harsh, and to quietly set about the task of reconciling oneself to it. The difference was between parents who laid down draconian rules about drinking and smoking, and parents who were "cool" — they knew it happened, it was the way of the world, they accepted it. So, like Baranoski and her fellow researchers, I was surprised at the results of their study. Patients who ranted and raved, it seemed to me, would be as likely to improve the outcome of their disease as parents in denial would be likely to change their kids' behavior.

But what Baranoski's study showed was that there are actually two kinds of denial. First, there's the classic form of denial: "I'm not sick" or "I know I'm sick, but I'm not going to let this disease interfere with my life." I spoke to one patient whose advice to other cancer patients was this: "Just put it out of your mind that anything can hurt you. Just go through there [the hospital] like nothing could possibly hurt you. Enjoy yourself, and that's it." Another patient, after a close brush with death due to a burst AVM (arteriovenous malformation), bragged, "To this day, if you ask me what those initials are, AVM — is that it? — I can't re-member what they stand for. And I don't want to." *That* is classic denial.

But there's another kind of denial. It is, paradoxically, an *affirm-ing* denial, a denial that's not about "what I won't do" (I won't let this disease get to me), but about "what I *will* do" (I will do whatever I need to do to get better); a denial that says, "I know I'm sick, but I'm going to beat this thing." Another cancer pa-tient described his attitude this way: "I just made up my mind *that with the help of my wife, we were going to go step by step and lick it.*" As Baranoski points out, this kind of denial can take many forms. For Alice Trillin, it was solving a problem. For Gary Shields, the California college student with testicular cancer, it was playing to win. "I've always been a very competitive-type person," says Shields, "very competitive in sports, in academics, and in this. So I said, 'Let's go for it, let's do it.' Don't take no for an answer, just keep going."

That's *positive* denial. That's the kind of denial patients need, the kind of denial that makes it possible to carry on the fight. "There are people who fight to the last breath," says Dr. David Peretz, a psychiatrist who specializes in terminal illness and grief. "But to fight to the last breath you have to deny to the last breath. If you're not denying, then that in itself opens the door to another kind of experience: resignation. So denial is very, very useful both in keeping people fighting and probably in keeping the immune system going. I think that's why, when people with life-threatening illnesses really decide that they've had it, they die very soon. They die very soon once they let go."

What about prayer? I myself am not a religious person, but I have talked to many patients who believe that prayer, and prayer alone, made the difference between life and death for them. I have also heard about studies showing that when people prayed for half of the patients in an intensive care unit, that half had better recoveries — even when the patients *didn't know* someone was praying for them.

Kim Peay felt a strange pain in her neck and shoulders after the birth of her second child in 1991. Her local doctors thought it was nothing, and it wasn't until two years later, when she began falling down inexplicably, that she was diagnosed with a spinal cord tumor. By a stroke of good luck, she ended up in the office of Dr. Bennett Stein, *my* Bennett Stein, at Columbia-Presbyterian in New York. "I was real scared," Peay recalls. "When they told me it was a tumor, I thought, 'Oh, my gosh, I've got two children to raise.' But all the time I felt like something was telling me, 'It's all right, don't worry, everything's going to be just fine.' I believe in miracles, too. I believe in the power of prayer." Not only did Peay pray, but her church back in Jonesville, South Carolina (my state), held a prayer vigil the night before her surgery. "We had so many people praying for me," says Peay, "I believe God just worked through Dr. Stein to save my life."

She was, indeed, saved. There was a scare immediately after the surgery when she was temporarily paralyzed, and she had to spend seven weeks in rehabilitation relearning how to walk, but today her tumor is "completely gone." "That sounds like a miracle to me," says Peay.

Perhaps. But no different from the other miracles that happen in hospital beds and operating rooms every day, I would argue. "It's true that patients who believe in a higher power tend to do better," says Dr. Nicholas Gonzalez, the alternative medicine guru who admits that "initially, I had trouble believing this." Why do they do better? "Prayer eliminates anxiety," Gonzalez explains. "Patients tend to turn over all their worries to a higher force. With God in charge, they can relax. The best relaxation technique I have found, and I have tried everything with patients from biofeedback to meditation, is prayer. Prayer just seems to work better than anything, and it doesn't matter whether it's Jewish, Christian, or Moslem. If they pray, they seem to do better. There are people at NIH now who are looking at prayer as a therapeutic tool."

But just as there are two kinds of denial, there are two kinds of prayer. Rhonda Kraemer, another patient of Dr. Stein's, was, like Kim Peay, a mother of two in her late twenties who was diagnosed with a fatal tumor. "My doctors told me, 'There's nothing we can do,'" she remembers, "and to plan the rest of my life because there wasn't much hope." Unwilling to take "nothing we can do" for an answer, Kraemer kept looking until she found Dr. Stein. After a series of embolizations and surgery, she, too, had an arduous recovery. She had to learn how to read again. She, too, found strength in her faith. "I had an inner survival instinct," she says, "an instinct to keep going, no matter what, to keep pushing on. And it was my God that gave me that. That's the truth. He gave me a desire to keep on living."

Rhonda Kraemer's faith in her God was like Alice Trillin's faith in her problem-solving skills or like Gary Shields's faith in his competitive prowess. It *empowered* her. It gave her faith in her *own* power to alter the course of her disease. It gave her strength for the struggle — "a desire to keep on living." It gave her a fighting spirit. Simple faith isn't enough. I talked to the relatives of another very religious patient who died within hours of deciding that "God was calling her home." According to Dr. Baranoski (who refers not to patients who believe in God, but to patients "whose hope is structured by their faith"), the only way to make "the belief in an external agent that is the source of one's power, one's hopefulness, and one's optimism truly *useful* is to move that faith into one's self." It isn't a matter of *what* the patient has faith in, it's a matter of what that faith gives the patient. Dr. James Cimino, a nephrologist at Calvary Hospital in the Bronx, told me about a study "where they tried to determine whether or not people who have the will to live do better. What they found is that *where that will to live leads you to* do *things,* it can make a difference," says Cimino. "But the beneficial effects of wishful thinking and prayer alone are very difficult to prove."

That's what "positive denial" and "positive prayer" have in common — they "lead you to *do* things." While attitude is undoubtedly important, it has to be accompanied by actions — both the patient's and the doctor's. The right doctor performing the right treatment on a patient with the right attitude is how medical miracles like Kim Peay's *and* Alice Trillin's happen. "I don't think somebody by a sheer act of will has a miraculous healing process where all their metastases disappear," says Dr. Andrew von Eschenbach, the urologic surgeon. "Nor do I think we ought to attribute it just to the fact that the therapy was miraculous or the drug was miraculous. The miracle is in the interaction between the two — the patients' efforts, both mental and actual, and the right therapy. It's the patients' spirit and the patients' vitality and their willingness to endure and overcome and survive that, combined with the therapy we offer, seems to have a miraculous effect; that is, an outcome that surpasses the odds of what you would have expected."

Prayer by itself isn't enough, faith isn't enough, optimism isn't enough, even the will to live, by itself, no matter how strong, isn't enough if you just sit back and let things happen. You have to *do* something. But what? Every doctor I spoke to agreed — after all the options have been pursued, all the treatments weighed, the balance struck and the best doctor chosen — patients need to do something to *affirm* their lives. They use different terms — Dr. Klagsbrun, the psychiatrist, calls it "investing in living";

Dr. Hannah Hedrick, an official of the American Medical Association, calls it "conscious living"; Thomas Petty, the pulmonologist, "building on today"— but it all amounts to the same thing. "We're talking about *sustaining a claim to life*," says Dr. Peretz, "in a healthy and appropriate way."

That way can be as simple as setting goals: finish this, see that, do this. For one patient I spoke to, it was a daughter's graduation; for another, a son's marriage. "There are elderly people that come in and are taking this thing in their own hands," says Dr. W. Marston Linehan, "and I've often heard elderly patients come in here and say, I want to see my grandkids, so I am going to do what I have to do to kick this."

A seventy-year-old Texas man came to Dr. Petty's office in Denver saying that he had been given two years to live by a well-known pulmonologist in Dallas. "Today's my birthday," the man said. "My two years are up today."

"Well, isn't it good that you came on your birthday," said Petty, "because let's just plan for two more birthdays." He asked the man what he wanted to do in the next two years.

"I want to see my first grandson born," the man said.

Two years later, that man was in the hospital waiting room when his grandson was delivered by C-section exactly on his grandfather's birthday, the second anniversary of his visit to Petty. "That way," says Petty, "every time he celebrated his birthday, he celebrated his grandson's birthday — and his own survival."

Soon after his grandson's birth, the man came to see Petty again. "So what do you want to do now?" Petty asked.

"I want to reach eighty," he said.

"The last time I looked, he was seventy-nine," says Petty. "He uses a wheelchair more now, but he can still walk. I myself am amazed that he's still alive."

Other patients "sustain their claim to life" by joining self-help or support groups. "That's a way of making a *commitment to living* rather than struggling against death," says the AMA's

Dr. Hedrick, who conducts therapy groups for AIDS patients. "These groups save lives. A patient comes in who literally might have been planning to commit suicide — because of isolation or despair — and he sees all these people who have been living with the disease for ten years, and are funny and happy and healthy and dancing, and it changes him. It transforms him on the spot. That's very thrilling. It's also very good for his immune system."

Other patients "sustain their claim to life" by concentrating on living their own lives *better*. Dr. Klagsbrun tells about a patient, a divorcée with three children who, when she was diagnosed with very advanced Hodgkin's disease, quit her job as an editor and concentrated on her long-secret desire to write. Then she met a man "who was profoundly in love with her," according to Klagsbrun, "and good to her kids, and desperately wanted to marry her. She loved him, too, but said she didn't want to make a widower out of him."

When she brought her dilemma to the support group that Klagsbrun led, the group members wanted to know "Why are you preparing for death? Why not invest that energy in anticipating living so that you can live a better life?" The group took a vote. They voted that she should go home that very night and propose to the man. "She did," says Klagsbrun. "And he accepted. They married and she's still alive. They're still happily together." They send Klagsbrun a card every Christmas. "I don't want to say that she was cured because she changed her life," says Klagsbrun. "She was forced to confront the quality of her life and she did something about it. To the extent that had some positive beneficial influence on her disease, so be it."

Harold Taylor, as usual, is eloquent on the subject of using illness as a prism to reexamine one's life. "I think it's quite important for people who are sick to ask themselves: How seriously are you treating yourself? How far are you prepared to go in giving yourself the best chance of getting better? Are you still drinking heavily or still smoking? How responsible are you being to yourself? People must *examine the whole way in which they conduct their lives.*"

Patients like Klagsbrun's divorcée and Harold Taylor see illness not just as a warning, not just as a battle, but as an opportunity. Taylor told me about another patient he knew, a young man who had been to a prestigious business school and was working on Wall Street, but was "really unhappy, really conflicted; didn't think it was for him, but didn't know how to get out of it." Then he was diagnosed with colon cancer. After a long, arduous course of treatment, the young man decided to go back to school and get a master's degree in teaching. "Today he is teaching in an inner-city school," says Taylor, "and he's truly happy. It was only the fact that he got this dread disease and could have died that made him say, 'What the hell am I doing?'"

That's a patient who didn't just "sustain his claim to life," he staked a deeper claim. "I certainly don't wish cancer on anybody," says Taylor. "But I do think that for many people, it does provide them with some good."

Alice Trillin would go further than that. "One of the gratifying things about getting sick," she says, "one of the truly positive things about getting sick for a lot of people, is that they find out that they can do things that they never thought they could do."

Dr. Linehan remembers a patient of his, a woman his own age, who had a "very difficult disease," kidney cancer, but also a tenacious grip on life. "Her cancer had spread," he recalls, "and it was very serious." When he walked into her hospital room to discuss her treatment, she was on the phone. "Oh, I'll be off in just a minute," she told him. "She was talking to her daughter," Linehan recalls, "and saying things like, 'Okay, now look, tomorrow wear the gray sweater and make sure that your brother gets his homework done. Mommie is going to be home soon. You guys don't worry, and make sure that your little sister gets her report done for Monday.'"

Linehan thought about his own daughters. "As I listened to

her," he recalls, "I was thinking to myself: This is such a serious disease. You certainly hope that a patient like this will be cured of her disease, but more often than not, that's not the case. We are talking about kidney cancer, a very tough killer. Once the disease has spread, only ten to twenty percent of patients typically survive two years.

"So I'm listening to this lady talk to her kids, and I'm thinking what could potentially be down the line in this lady's future, and I think to myself: You've just got to fight back the tears, be upbeat here, keep on working. It's just incomprehensible how much courage some of these people have. It makes it so I don't want to go home at night. You tell yourself you've just got to work harder. You've got to work faster. You've got to do better."

FOURTEEN

Beating the System

WHAT WAS I thinking about as I looked forward to my second major brain surgery in a decade? Would I be able to write afterward? Would I lose some memory? How much, and which ones? Would I be plunged back into the hermitage of facial paralysis? How visible would the scar be? Would my hair grow back? Would I live past forty?

All these questions, and more, floated through my head as I waited for the day in April 1992 when the operation with Dr. Dolenc was scheduled. But the question that overrode all of them, that dogged me morning, noon, and night, and kept me awake till dawn, wasn't any of these. It wasn't one of the "big questions" about life and death: things I wished I had done but hadn't, or things I had done but wished I hadn't. No, this question was about *money*. In particular, where would I get the money to pay for this operation?

Before, I had always been one of the lucky ones. As a student at Harvard, I had insurance. As a television writer in Los Angeles, I had insurance. Indeed, I had paid only a small deductible, $800 I believe, out of all the expenses related to my first big surgery at U.C.L.A. After that, I went on my father's small-business policy for a while, but because of the size of his business and my medical history, the premiums went up like a bottle rocket and he was forced to "spin me off" into an individual policy with more fine print than a car rental agreement. Even with my legal training, I couldn't actually tell by reading the policy if the operation with Dr. Dolenc would be covered. Would they consider his pathbreaking cavernous sinus surgery "non-standard therapy"? Or my persistent tumor a "pre-existing condition?" If so, someone else would have to pay the $100,000 plus bill — on a writer's income, I certainly couldn't — or, of course, I could forgo the operation. And then what?

My dilemma was hardly unique. One of the saddest things about the American medical system is that the most desperately ill often have to fight the hardest to pay their bills. A patient who is already fighting to find a last-ditch treatment — any treatment — when all standard therapies have failed, may not be able to pay for that treatment when and if he finds it. And, as my case shows, it's not just a problem for the poor and the uninsured. Whether the source of payment is an HMO, an insurance company, or a federal program like Medicaid, the stone wall of resistance is the same.

A lucky few, of course, are spared this salt-on-the-wound battle. I talked to several patients who lived every patient's dream of hassle-free payment. Max Marsh was in New Orleans when doctors discovered a large mass between his heart and lung. Only one doctor could safely remove the tumor, the world-renowned tracheal surgeon, Hermes Grillo. But Dr. Grillo was in Boston, at the Massachusetts General Hospital. "I went to my insurance company," says Marsh, "and they said, 'Mr. Marsh, we'll let you go anywhere you want in the world.'" And their response when he told them he wanted the surgery done by Dr. Grillo at M.G.H.? "They said, 'Mr. Marsh, you made the best decision you ever made in your life.'"

But for every patient like Max Marsh with a gilt-edged insurance policy, there are ten patients, like me, for whom the issue of who pays the bills is not a dream but a nightmare. The same Dr. Grillo told me about another patient of his, a teacher, who had a tracheal tumor and whose local doctors had told him there was nothing that could be done surgically. His only recourse was radiation. But this man did his homework and found Dr. Grillo, who examined him and concluded that his tumor was "perfectly manageable surgically with a good potential for cure." But when the man returned to his home state and talked to his insurance company, he hit the stone wall. "They told him if he wanted to get on a plane for treatment," Grillo recalls, "he would have to pay forty percent of the cost himself — which was the same as saying no, because he was on a teacher's salary."

"But you can't offer me this treatment at home," the man complained to his insurance company.

"We are offering you *a* treatment," they said. "Radiation."

"But that's inevitably going to lead to my death," he said.

"Well, *that's your problem*," they said. "Technically, the plan says you're going out of state and therefore you pay forty percent. Period."

That man ended up not coming to M.G.H. because, says Grillo, "like a damn fool, he put the costs above his care, and he'll die as a result."

Whatever the outcome, insurance battles like that put patients through a hell of uncertainty, a hell that the desperately ill (and their immune systems), already under stress, can hardly afford. I spoke to two patients who ultimately won their fight for coverage, but paid a high price. One, when told by her doctor that the lung surgery she needed would cost "in the six-figure category," spent six long weeks waiting for an answer from her insurance company, all the time thinking, "Well, do I give up everything I have to try to save my life and come out of it with nothing?" The other began a series of last-ditch experimental cancer treatments, each of which

191

took seventeen days in the hospital and cost about $20,000, but was told by his company after the first treatment, "We won't pay for it." "So I had a lot of stress, mental stress, just thinking about the finances of it all," recalls John Romney, a phone company employee in rural Tennessee, "the house, the car, the kids in college, and wondering if this treatment was going to have to come to a stop since maybe it wouldn't work in the first place."

The fundamental problem here, of course, is that insurance companies and the like are only interested in one thing: money. "Their primary goal is to retain funds as long as possible," says Dr. John Marini, the pulmonary and critical care specialist at St. Paul – Ramsey Medical Center, "and *not* spend money on patients." Unfortunately, one of the easiest strategies for not spending money is to deny payment for "experimental" procedures and protocols — which, in the case of rare diseases or intractable problems, is the same as denying payment altogether. "The insurance companies are, most of the time, interested only in money," says Dr. Grillo, "not patients. They don't even really claim to be health providers. They're just money managers."

And who decides what's "experimental" and what's not?

The insurance companies, of course. "They just love to call something experimental," says Grillo, who has had his share of battles with insurers, "because then they don't have to pay for it." Grillo tells the story of a patient who came to him from California with a very rare disease — so rare, in fact, that he had only operated on one previous case in all his years of doing airway surgery. Still, Grillo *devised* a new procedure for the problem, performed it, and the patient recovered well. Everybody was happy.

Except the insurance company. They wouldn't pay for the procedure. "It's experimental," they said.

"But we have a patient who's been cured," Grillo argued.

"It's experimental," they said.

"But it was this man's only hope," Grillo argued.

"It's experimental," they said.

"It's a unique solution to a unique problem," Grillo replied. "It's a rare case, and if you want to wait for a series of cases, you'll have to wait *a thousand years.*"

"It's experimental," they said.

Usefulness, success, hope, uniqueness, survival — none of these mean much to a bunch of money managers trying to keep costs down. What they want is standardization and predictability, and they have devised myriad ways, some of them devilishly clever, of achieving it, putting roadblocks in the way of doctors whose treatments are unstandardized and patients whose diseases are unpredictable, and complicating life even further for everyone working at the edges of the possible to make miracles happen.

Denying payment is only the most direct way in which insurers can discourage nonstandard treatments. They can get much the same effect, without risking legal liability or moral indignation, by *agreeing* to pay —*just not very much.* That way, doctors have less (monetary) incentive to offer them. Dr. Robert Brumback, the trauma surgeon, told me about a patient he called "the lady of stone." As the result of a bad car accident, the woman suffered serious liver, lung, and spinal cord damage. After six weeks on a respirator, she began to develop heterotopic ossification, or "bone out of place." Her bones began to fuse at the joints: first her shoulders, then her elbows, then both hips and both knees. Before long, she couldn't walk. Eventually, frozen permanently in a semi-seated position, she couldn't move at all. Only her wrists still functioned. She ate with an eighteen-inch fork, and when she answered the phone, she had to shout to cover the two feet from her hand to her mouth. She had been in that position for more than a year when she found Dr. Brumback.

In two massive operations, Brumback resected the heterotopic ossification from around every major joint of her body. Eight in all. In each operation, he did the shoulder and elbow on one side and the hip and knee on the other. In many places, the errant bone had grown around arteries and nerves, making the surgery both extraordinarily arduous and exceedingly delicate. Each operation took twelve hours. Brumback billed Blue Cross/Blue Shield $8,000 for each twelve-hour day of surgery, a total charge of $16,000. The insurer mailed him a check for $5,000.

"I know there are a lot of people for whom twenty-five hundred dollars a day is a ton of money," says Brumback, "an absolute ton, and I'm very sensitive to that issue." Yet, on one of the days between the two surgeries on the lady of stone, Brumback did a routine arthroscopy procedure on another patient. "I just looked inside his knee, found some loose bodies floating around in there, and kind of shaved the cartilage a bit." For that, Brumback submitted a bill for $4,000 and the insurance company paid him $3,100. "So for an hour and a half's work on that guy, I got thirty-one hundred dollars, but for twelve hours on this poor lady, I got twenty-five hundred." *That's* the problem, says Brumback. "There's no rhyme or reason to these insurance numbers. But I can tell you one thing: There is no reimbursement and no recognition for the difficulty of the case."

Insurers can also discourage doctors by forcing them to jump through bureaucratic hoops, hoops that are sometimes degrading, often unnecessary, occasionally idiotic, and always frustrating. "I get awfully tired of being jerked around," says Dr. John Marini. "Do you know what I have to do to write a prescription that some jackass functionary, working for an insurance company, working from a list, tells me I have to do if I want to prescribe a medication that's off the formulary, but is particularly useful? I have to call them and get permission from somebody who doesn't know anything about medicine or, even if they're a doctor, doesn't know the patient, doesn't know me, doesn't know my specialty, doesn't know anything except how to throw roadblocks in the way so I don't prescribe medicines that they don't want to pay for."

Dr. Grillo at M.G.H. had a patient with histoplasmosis, an infectious disease similar to tuberculosis. She was coughing up blood, having progressively greater difficulty breathing, and, according to

Grillo, "was going to die." The doctors in her midwestern home-town knew she needed an operation, "but weren't willing to touch it." So, like a lot of difficult thoracic patients, she ended up in Dr. Grillo's operating room at M.G.H. — for ten and a half hours. "It was a very tough surgery," Grillo recalls, "but we got it out and didn't have to take any lung out. Fortunately, she did well and went home."

Unfortunately, that wasn't the end of the story. Because she was a Medicare patient, the Commonwealth of Massachusetts paid Grillo "the usual pathetic amount. I think it came out to something like thirteen hundred dollars for everything: surgery, postoperative care, preoperative care, the works." And because Massachusetts hospitals are not allowed to bill patients for any balance due, that was the *whole* fee: thirteen hundred dollars.

It was the patient's husband, not Grillo, who considered that amount "outrageous" and wrote a strong letter of protest to Massachusetts Medicare. After a long wait, he received a reply, which he showed to Grillo. "It said, 'Our skilled reviewers have gone over the amount paid, and we find it to be perfectly appro-priate,'" Grillo recalls, "which, of course, was perfectly ridiculous because there was nobody else in Massachusetts doing this except us. Then it said, 'You should know that this is unnecessary surgery and therefore if you paid any amounts to the above provider' — not doctor, provider, that really gravels me — 'here's the proce-dure for *getting your money back*'!"

But that wasn't all. To add insult to injury, it went on to give Grillo's patient some gratuitous advice. "You should know that we have had trouble with this Hermes Grill [*sic*] in the past, in that he's done this unnecessary surgery before." *That,* much more than the pathetic reimbursement, made Grillo furious. "So some clerk in Hingham is deciding what's necessary and unnecessary surgery?" he fumed. "And what's their definition of unnecessary surgery? Their definition of unnecessary is that it's not on their list of standard procedures." After writing a scathing letter, Grillo received a check for an additional $200 in reimbursement. Grillo's angry response: "That was just exactly *not* the issue."

Another favorite strategy insurance companies use to avoid paying for experimental procedures (and thereby discourage them) is a cynical combination of ignorance and delay. One doctor, a cancer specialist, explained it to me this way (off the record): "The insurer says no to everybody and acts like they have never heard of the treatment before, like 'Oh, gee, that's a novel idea. Please have your doctor go through all the paperwork on that and send it in and we'll decide if we want to pay for it or not.' When, in fact, that same insurance company said the same thing last month, last year; has asked that same question twenty times as a delaying strategy specifically to slow the process down. They know the patient is dying, and dying over a few months, and the more they can slow the process, the fewer patients they will have to pay for.

"Now occasionally, when the aggressive patient or the aggressive doctor really presses them, they will often say, 'Okay, we're going to do this with you,' and they open the gate a bit and let *that* patient through. He or she gets the experimental procedure paid for. But then the next patient wants in that same gate a few minutes later and they say, 'Oh, gee, that's a new procedure. We don't know what to think about that.'" Because there is no clearinghouse for information about what treatments have been accepted elsewhere for reimbursement — what patients have been "let through the gate" — it's easy for insurance companies to get away with stonewalling.

As disturbing as tight money can be to a patient who, like me, is looking for the best medical care, even more disturbing is the effect the reimbursement system has on the quality of care. More and more, insurance companies and HMOs are making it difficult not just to pay for the best care, but to *seek* the best care. And even, in a few cases, to *get* the best care. "It doesn't take a rocket scientist," says Dr. James Kirklin, "to figure out that if you're an insurance company and you want to make money on a patient, you let 'em die on the first day."

No one thinks that we have sunk that low, but every doctor I spoke to agreed that we are, indeed, sinking in that direction. Hospitals will not stop treating patients just because they don't have insurance or their insurance runs out. Indeed, most states have laws that require emergency rooms to admit patients without a "wallet biopsy," as it is called, and forbid them from dumping uninsured patients on other hospitals. "But," says a prominent trauma surgeon, "off the record, these financial considerations enter into patient care more and more these days, especially when you're providing expensive, cutting-edge care and there is maybe a fifteen to twenty percent chance of recovery. It accelerates the whole pace of decision making. The harsh reality is that, especially in some institutions, treatment is going to be cut short because of financial considerations if the patient is not adequately insured."

For patients who, like me, fall below that "fifteen to twenty percent" cut-off, that is, indeed, an ominous development.

So what can patients do? How can they fight an increasingly restrictive, oppressive system? "The first thing," according to Dr. Marini, "is to know the consequences of not being adequately insured. It can be fabulously expensive." Even someone who is insured may not be *adequately* insured. Policies that cover regular checkups and occasional minor problems may crumble under the weight of a catastrophic illness and an all-out search for the best medical care. "It used to be that all you needed was a second opinion and the insurance company would follow you to a place like M.G.H.," says Dr. Grillo, "that and the wherewithal to go to Boston was all you needed." Even now, with a really good policy, like Max Marsh's, that's all a patient needs. But without that kind of gilt-edged policy, most patients who want the best treatment will, sooner or later, have to fight.

And, sooner or later, they will need an advocate.

Some patients, of course, have the disposition, the resources, the training, the chutzpah, the whatever, to be their own advocates. That's how I solved my dilemma. After waiting until after the surgery, when the insurance company did indeed refuse to pay for Dolenc's "experimental procedure," I mounted a full-scale appeal, putting on my seldom-worn lawyer's hat, and writing a stern "to whom it may concern" letter that included dark references to "legal precedents" and "what a jury would think" and signing it "Gregory W. Smith, *Esq.*" The company agreed to "revisit" my claim and eventually approved almost full reimbursement. More often than not, however, mounting and maintaining a drawn-out battle like that against an entrenched bureaucracy requires more energy, more frustration, and especially more time than a seriously ill patient can afford.

Fortunately, most of the doctors I spoke to — especially those who deal with seriously ill patients and experimental treatments — are eager to lend their energy and expertise to the battle. "That is something I do literally every single day," says a prominent cancer specialist. "A patient comes in here for treatment and the insurance company doesn't want to pay. I write letters for patients all the time. We have to press very hard to get insurers to do things, including our government insurance programs. That's a constant problem." Dr. Grillo, who has written many letters to his patients' insurers, believes that "with a letter from a really aggressive physician who is interested in the patient, you can push insurers into agreeing. The problem is that the system puts people who are not aggressive or sophisticated at a terrible disadvantage. The average person out there doesn't play tough with the insurance company. They don't know they can. That's why they need an advocate."

Sometimes, of course, patients need more advocacy than even the most aggressive doctor can give them. Sometimes, they need a lawyer. Lawyers have the two things that patients need most: information and credibility. As my experience shows, there is nothing like the threat of a lawsuit to get an insurer to "revisit" a request for reimbursement. Dr. Grillo tells the story of a patient with a very aggressive cancer of the lung who found an experimental treatment at Memorial Sloan-Kettering that offered her "a thirty percent chance of cure where otherwise it was zero," according to Grillo. "But her HMO said, 'No, we're not going to send you there. It costs too much money.'" But this woman had one advantage many patients don't: Her son was a lawyer. "He went to work on it and the HMO agreed to review the case and they changed their minds," says Grillo. "They didn't want a lawsuit."

Why didn't they want a lawsuit? Because lawsuits leave records — *public* records, which other patients can see. If they settle, as they did in this woman's case, there doesn't have to be a public record, and usually isn't. Indeed, insurers often demand as a condition of settlement that the patient not divulge any information about the reimbursement. That way, when the next patient comes "to the gate" with the same request, the company can say, "Oh, gee, that's a new treatment. We don't pay for that."

Because there is no clearinghouse for data on what treatments have been accepted by what insurers for reimbursement, often the *only* way to find such information is by consulting lawyers who have handled similar cases in the past. "If you have access to the information that a claim like yours has already been paid for through an insurance company," says the cancer specialist, who routinely puts his patients in touch with lawyers to help them fight insurance companies, "obviously you are in much better shape. Then you can go to them and say, 'Wait a second, you already paid for so-and-so's operation.' But the only way to get access to that information is through the lawyers who specialize in that kind of information. There is no group or institution that really helps patients get that information."

One doctor I spoke to envisioned a day when patients who have been turned down by their insurance companies will be able to pick up the phone and dial 1-800-MED-HELP and find out, "Yes, there have been twenty-eight cases just like yours. Here is the list of them and here are the lawyers who handled those cases and their phone numbers. Get this information to your insurance company and they will fold in three minutes." Dr. Grillo expects that, sooner or later, a new specialty will develop in the law: forcing HMOs to pay for appropriate treatment. "Lawyers will advertise for clients. Like the signs on the Boston subway saying, 'Does your baby have a birth defect? Perhaps your doctor was to blame.' Only these signs will say, 'Are you unable to get the care you need? Call attorney so-and-so.'"

Until that day, though, patients will have to continue to rely primarily on the efforts of doctor/advocates like Joel Cooper. As a surgeon specializing in pathbreaking transplant procedures, Cooper has had more than his share of battles with insurers. In particular, he has challenged their insistence on waiting until an experimental procedure is published in the literature before they will approve it. "That automatically gives them about three years to stall," he says, "even though there's a *proven benefit*." He tells insurers, "It's your obligation to get *current* information, and the current information comes from the doctor, and that's me."

Of Cooper's many battles with insurance companies, none was more fierce than the one over his second double lung transplant. The first was done on Ann Harrison and the Canadian health system paid for it, but the second patient's insurer, Blue Cross/Blue Shield, balked. They would pay for a heart/lung transplant because that was an established procedure, but not for this new experimental double lung transplant. Cooper tried to explain to them that he wouldn't know until he was in the operating room if he would do the double lung transplant or the more traditional heart/lung operation (in which both the patient's lungs and heart are removed and the donor's heart and lungs, still attached to each other, are put in). "If we feel we can leave the patient's heart in," Cooper explained, "we will cut the heart off of the donor specimen and put in just the two lungs." That way, the patient would get to keep her own heart and the donor heart could be used for another patient.

Blue Cross/Blue Shield was unmoved: "We cover heart/lung transplants," they repeated, "but not double lung transplants."

"Wait a minute," said Cooper. "Let me get this straight. I go in the operating room. I have in the bucket a heart and two lungs. I have in the patient a heart and two lungs. If I cut the heart *and* the lungs out of the patient, we get paid everything. But if I leave the heart *in* and just put in the two lungs, we get nothing. Right?"

Right.

"So you want me to go into the operating room and make a decision about what I think is best for that patient, knowing that if I decide to put in the heart *and* the lungs, the hospital collects for everything, but if I decide — for the good of the patient — to put in just the two lungs, then it's nothing. Are you sure that's what you want?"

When the company still wouldn't budge, the patient's husband informed the papers in Boston, his hometown, of the dispute and one of them sent a reporter to interview Cooper. "I asked all the same questions on the front page," Cooper recalls. He also pointed out that the double lung transplant he proposed used a small piece of the donor heart (although not enough to preclude the use of the rest of the organ for another transplant). "So I asked on the front page of the Boston paper, 'How much heart has to be left on the lung in order to be paid by Blue Cross/Blue Shield? Does it have to be the whole heart or half a heart? Is a quarter of a heart enough?'"

Only a short time after the article appeared, Cooper received a letter from Blue Cross/Blue Shield; they were "reviewing" his application. "I knew we were getting somewhere," says Cooper, "because they started referring to her operation as the 'double lung/partial heart transplant.'"

Eventually, after the operation, Cooper went to Boston to plead his patient's case to Blue Cross/Blue Shield in person. At the end of the hearing, he introduced the examiners to the patient herself. "I snuck her in without them knowing it," he recalls, "and brought her out so they could see how well she was doing." The company approved the operation, and the patient — only the second in the world — "is eight years post-op and doing wonderfully," according to Cooper. "Hasn't had a problem at all."

Since that hearing, Cooper has fought similar battles against other insurers, Medicare, and the Veterans Administration in twenty-six states, and *never lost a case*. Most of them, for all the reasons discussed above, never went to trial. "They would drag it out and drag it out," Cooper recalls, "then they would have a discovery, I'd give a deposition, and just before trial they would settle because they knew if they went to trial they would lose and they didn't want that as a matter of record. By settling the case, they could make the patient agree that he wouldn't sue. The company would pay the expenses, leaving itself in a position to deny coverage to the next patient."

But Cooper isn't resting. "I am actually starting the whole process over again now with the emphysema surgery," he says, referring to the experimental lung reduction surgery that Morton Silberman had. "Some insurance companies have covered it; some have not." And now he tells his emphysema patients the same thing he used to tell his transplant patients: "If your insurer refuses to pay, you get a lawyer and I'll back you up. If you can't afford a lawyer, the hospital will pay for one. And if you don't win, we won't charge you anything."

FIFTEEN

"Why Me?"

FINALLY, THE DAY came. I flew into Charlottesville, Virginia, on a small USAir plane in a clear but bumpy blue sky. Jefferson's magnificent campus with its domed library and long white colonnades lining an emerald rectangle of lawn appeared out of the rolling Shenandoah hills. A chaos of newer buildings "in the style of Jefferson" grew like a red brick cancer around this perfect center. At the edge of the cancer stood a tall, aluminum-clad modern building that I knew at first glance, even from a thousand feet up, was the hospital. Once I saw it, I couldn't take my eyes off it. As I stared, a question kept trying to form in my head — something like, "If I go in there, will I ever come out?" — but I wouldn't let it.

Just as I wouldn't let the beautiful spring weather lift my spirits. In the seven months since my fateful post-Pulitzer meeting with Dr. Hilal, I had fought the self-flagellating urge to see an ill omen in every cloudy day or unreturned phone call. I wasn't about to start now, even for a *good* omen, even for the sake of a little uplift on the eve of my surgery. For good or ill, superstition was superstition. Still, as the plane repeatedly circled the town—some trouble on the ground; I didn't want to think about it—I had more time for thoughts than I would have wanted.

For seven months, I had been fighting a daily battle *with myself.* A mental battle. Not paying attention to "signs" was just a part of that battle: probably the easiest part. I had gotten past the fear — the plain, old-fashioned, garden-variety fear — the involuntary rush of dire hypotheticals and grim imaginings that used to surprise me in the middle of the night: What if my face is paralyzed? What if I lose my eye? My memory? Will I be able to write? Will I die? I had even gotten past the fear of pain, for the most part. No, the mental battle that still raged even as we circled over the Virginia hills, and the April sunlight lanced in one side of the plane and then the other, wasn't with any enemy as ennobling as fear.

The enemy now — the only enemy left, in fact — was the enemy within.

It was the enemy I met every time I walked down the street, went to a movie, or sat in a restaurant, and had to fight the urge to envy everyone around me, everyone with "normal" lives, "normal" health, "normal" futures. What did they do to deserve that flawlessness? Then, in my dreams, the envy would come flooding out. In the old days, when my bones were disintegrating and I couldn't breathe or walk without pain, I used to dream of running and jumping. Now I dreamed only of being normal again. (Only once did I dream of the tumor. It began to ooze out my ear, then the ooze turned to a jet, like a sprung leak, of thick shiny liquid the consistency of motor oil.)

I found myself fascinated by babies. I would stare at their hairless heads and think, "How pure, how perfect, how *normal.* What a wonderful thing a normal head is, a head the way nature made it. *I* once had a head like that." I would study baby pictures of myself looking for . . . what? . . . a clue? a "sign"? some hint of disease? — and think, "If only I had known then what I know now, I would have appreciated that head more." And then, inevitably, I would scold myself for living a cliché. More than anything else, I hated becoming a cliché: the cliché of sickness, the cliché of despair, even the cliché of death: clichés within clichés.

But now, as the plane began to make its final approach, I could feel my life descending yet again into cliché. I thought about all those normal people down there, the healthy masses, the tumorless crowds. Even the green hills taunted me with their normality. The green of spring, the turning of seasons, the cycle of life — somehow I had been ejected from that cycle, rejected, like a flawed cog in the engine of life, estranged from everything normal. Permanently on the outside looking in. And maybe not even permanently.

Feeling sorry for myself? You bet. And why not? At least on one level, it seemed perfectly understandable, perfectly reasonable that I was feeling sorry for myself. I had a *brain tumor.* My life was in a state of ruinous upheaval as well as ruinous uncertainty; my family was in tears; my finances, my work, my life, in jeopardy. What's not to feel sorry for?

And the question that kept breaking through, no matter how hard I tried to beat it back, the question that seemed to lie at the end of every wild tangent of resentment or paranoia or anger or envy or despair, was the biggest cliché of all: "Why me?"

It is one of the many subtle cruelties of serious illness that after fighting for better care, fighting for more options, fighting mainstream medicine, and fighting insurance companies, many patients have to confront a still more formidable, final enemy: themselves.

That enemy can take the form of pessimism or resignation; it can be abetted by loved ones or even by doctors, although it is formidable with or without allies. It is every bit as hard to fight one's own impatience as to fight the intransigence of hospital and corporate bureaucracies; as difficult to overcome one's own frustration as the pessimism of doctors. But for many patients, the worst enemy of all is self-pity, the feelings of "Why me?" and "Poor me!" and the depression that inevitably follows in their wake.

There's a reason, of course, that "Why me?" is such a cliché: Almost every patient feels it, at some time to some degree. In many cases, like mine, the feeling can be aggravated by other factors like financial woes, family problems, or the effects of drugs. Even a patient's level of education can affect his or her vulnerability to this most corrosive of rhetorical questions. "When you're dealing with people intellectually above the norm," says Dr. Morton Silberman, the assistant director of the Woodruff Health Sciences Center at Emory, "they tend to think, 'I'm educated, I've been to graduate school, I'm so goddamned smart. I'm such a valuable person. *Why me?*' The arrogance sort of works to their disadvantage in a way, and they become more self-pitying."

The problem is that feelings of self-pity — why me, poor me — are the doorway to surrender, despondency, and even, in extreme cases, suicide. "That kind of attitude leads to an exaggerated perception of one's problems, a tunnel vision," says Dr. David Peretz, the psychiatrist. "Patients like that see things through a very narrow perspective, and that narrow perspective leaves out all the things that enable someone to fight." Harold Taylor saw the trap in self-pity. "I knew the 'why me' mentality would be hurtful to my chances," he recalls. "It would serve no purpose at all. Therefore, it was to be abandoned and rejected and kept at bay." If he sounds defensive, it's because even strong, self-assured patients like Harold Taylor — or (I thought) like me — are susceptible to the siren call of "Why me?"

Phyllis Forbes Kerr heard that call in 1966 when she was a twenty-three-year-old schoolteacher in Boston and her gynecologist felt "a mass" in her pelvic region. He rushed her into surgery the next day and "just reached in there and grabbed whatever it was," Kerr recalls. She heard the call again when "it" turned out to be, not the ectopic pregnancy her gynecologist had supposed, but cancer — and again when she learned that his hasty grab had spilled cancer cells all along its path: bladder, intestines, vagina. "In those days," she recalls, "when someone told you you had cancer, it was like you died right then." The gynecologist who did the surgery certainly thought so. He came in afterward and said he was sorry but, yes, it was cancer and, no, there was nothing that could be done about it. "Do you mean she's going to die?" Kerr's husband asked. "Yes," the doctor said.

No one, not even her family, disagreed. "It would be best for her mom if Phyllis doesn't linger," said Kerr's stepfather. "So the sooner she dies, the better." Her mother, whose sister had died at a young age, too, believed the doctor "was God Almighty," Kerr remembers, "so if the doctor was throwing up his hands, then the only polite thing to do was throw up her hands, too." Even Kerr's husband joined the chorus of despair. "He not only thought I was going to die," Kerr recalls, "he thought he might catch cancer from me."

But still Kerr never asked, "Why me?" Despite the despondency all around her and the insistent temptation to self-pity, she "just thought it was a great big pain in the neck." "I was going to live," says Kerr. "I was not going to give in to the pessimism. I was a brick." With the help of her husband, she found a surgeon, Dr. Lang Parsons, who did some creative cutting and managed both to save her reproductive organs and to build her a new bladder out of intestines (which meant she wouldn't have to wear a urine sack the rest of her life). In Kerr's book, being alive at all felt like a resounding victory.

A year and a half later, though, she heard the siren call again. An x-ray revealed nodules of cancer everywhere in her midsection — the legacy of her first doctor's hasty grab — too many for surgery. So she soldiered through a long, lonely regimen of radiation (when radiation was still in its crude infancy), a regimen that left her sick with massive diarrhea, torrential sweats, whiplash mood swings, heat flashes like solar flares and all the myriad miseries of premature menopause at age twenty-eight. But still she ignored the call. "I told myself, you've got to look at the big picture. This could be six operations." She even managed to ignore the call when they told her that because of the radiation she would never have children. Then when she and her husband decided to adopt, the adoption agencies gave them trouble over her health. *They* didn't think she would survive, either.

It wasn't too many years before she heard the call yet again. The doctors found a lump on her back and soon were saying that the tumor had metastasized to her liver. They were saying something else, too: that liver cancer was a disease hardly anybody survived. Kerr called her mother. "I think it's D-Day here," she joked blackly, "because I don't think you can operate on the liver."

"No," said her mother, characteristically upbeat, "I don't either."

She did, however, find a doctor who was willing to try. The only problem was that most of his previous liver operations had been unsuccessful. Most of the patients had bled to death on the table. It was a "very, very long shot," he told Kerr. He couldn't make any promises and had no idea what would happen. "I really think they all felt like I was going to die," Kerr recalls. And how did she feel? "I felt like Mary Queen of Scots on the way to the chopping block."

But still she refused to surrender to the call.

Even after the huge, day-long operation and the eternal agony of recovery — "I felt like I was tied to a railroad track, I felt pressure everywhere; it took two years before I could laugh without hurting" — she still refused to give in to self-pity. Through four more recurrences over twelve more years, with nodules as small as marbles and as big as grapefruit, with doctors saying *every time* that she was going to die, Phyllis Kerr refused to listen to the voice that whispered, "Why me?"

Then, on her sixth recurrence, twenty-five years after the first pain in her gut, she couldn't ignore the voice any longer. The liver cancer had come back and once again the doctors told her there was nothing they could do. This time, she *really* was going to die. The problem, they said, was that no doctor — not even the few who dared to operate on the liver at all — would operate on it a second time. The radiologist who first saw the recurrence on her scans couldn't even wait until she was dressed to bring her the bad news. "Chemotherapy, radiation, it doesn't really matter what you do," he said as she shivered in a hospital gown, "because you're going to die in a year or two anyway."

At first, Kerr was her usual defiant self. "I didn't believe him," she recalls. "I just did not believe him. And I was really mad because, I said to myself, the only thing I really have is hope, and he's trying to take that away from me." But by the time she got home, she was hearing a different voice. "I just thought, 'I can't do this. I just cannot do this,'" she remembers. "I thought, 'I've been through so much, and who needs any more?' I remember thinking, 'Why can't someone else do it? I've proved how strong I am and how brave and bold and all that stuff. I don't want to wish this on anybody else, but isn't it someone else's turn?'"

And then it was over. The next morning she woke up angry again, but not petulant or self-pitying. In twenty-five years, that was the closest she ever came to asking, "Why me?" the closest she ever came to surrendering. "But, you know, the days go by," she says, "and you just say, 'I'm going to do it.'" Fortunately for Phyllis Kerr, the radiologist turned out to be wrong: both about her and about the tumor. It wasn't in her liver, after all; it was in her diaphragm. Doctors removed a chunk of it, and she lived to see her adopted son turn twenty-four. And that makes her feel lucky, not unlucky. "I definitely take each day in a special way," she says, "treasure it more because of everything I've been through. It's made me see life another way."

Unfortunately, not every patient is as strong as Phyllis Kerr.

How does a patient who doesn't have Kerr's depth of conviction or inner strength or whatever — who isn't "a brick" — ignore the siren call of "Why me?" and steer clear of the rocky shores of self-pity, depression, and despair? The experts I spoke to — psychiatrists and support-group leaders who deal with seriously ill patients — all agree that the first step in breaking free of thoughts like the ones that followed me to the skies over Charlottesville is to understand *where they come from.*

For some people, self-pity comes out of depression. Everyone is depressed by bad news, of course. The question, according to Dr. William Wood, is "*Why* are they depressed?" For some, it's a "situational depression," says Wood. "These are the ones who say, 'Oh gosh, the tumor is back, I'm a goner. I just don't want to eat. I want to die. I don't want to face this. I'm going to throw in the towel.'" For patients like that, according to Wood, support groups, visits with other patients, and, of course, extra time and attention from a sympathetic doctor are often enough.

Other patients, however, have an "organic depression," says Wood, "something that they've battled all their lives," and they may need psychiatric help and medication to overcome it. "Very often these are people who feel a painful disappointment with their life in the present," says Dr. Peretz, "and the depression and self-pity they feel in response to that becomes displaced onto the illness." They bring a fatalism to all their endeavors, and catastrophic illness only gives that fatalism a new and poignantly literal twist. For them, the "Why me?" of illness just echoes the much wider and deeper "Why me?" of their failed lives.

According to Dr. Peretz, people like that are often in the grip of a "fate neurosis." "Everybody grows up with an idea of when they're going to die," he says, "which might be conditioned on when their parents died, or it may be connected with success. Some people believe that when they achieve success, they're going to be struck dead. There are lots of variations. People like that are inclined to give up, inclined not to push, inclined to believe that the worst outcome is unavoidable." Healthy people, on the other hand, people who are "enjoying their lives in the present," says

Peretz, "don't tend to give up when something like this comes along."

For some people, the self-pity of "Why me?" springs not from depression but from narcissism. Like Dr. Silberman's highly educated patients who consider themselves "so uniquely valuable" that their illness seems a special injustice, these people cannot reconcile disease with their self-image of achievement and perfection. For them, "Why me?" becomes "How could this happen to *me?*"

One day in the late 1980s on the Upper West Side of Manhattan where Steve and I used to live, a number of people were surprised to find a hand-delivered invitation under their door, an invitation unlike any they had ever received before. It was an invitation to a suicide. In it, a woman named Alice Sully, an artist in her mid-forties, announced that she had "terminal cancer" and that she was making a film about her dying. She was planning to make her death "a work of art," she said, and wanted her family, friends, and neighbors to participate.

Soon her story appeared on the front page of the *New York Times.* ("Not a bad place to get reviewed on your first performance," a friend quipped. "First and last.") Then PBS jumped on board with a program called "Choosing Suicide," in which Sully's film would be shown (posthumously, of course) and discussed by a panel of experts. Sully went through with her plan, gathering a group of friends around her bed for a farewell toast. They drank champagne. She drank hemlock.

After the suicide, but before the PBS show, however, one of the experts on the panel, a psychiatrist, decided to do some digging into Alice Sully's story. It turned out that she didn't have "terminal cancer" after all. All she had was a lump in her breast — with no metastases — and she had refused treatment for that. "She couldn't tolerate the injury to the view of herself that was entailed in the idea that she had cancer," says the psychiatrist. "She didn't have terminal cancer. She had terminal narcissism."

For some patients, the self-pity of "Why me?" is deeply rooted in masochism. For them, serious illness is just the final confirmation of their victimhood. "People with survival instincts [like Phyllis Kerr] see themselves as being caught with a temporary nuisance that they have to deal with," says Robert Knutzen, president of the Pituitary Tumor Society, and himself the survivor of a pituitary tumor with horrendous consequences, "and then there are others who go passively through life accepting that they are victims and must continue to be victims. The first group believes in themselves and believes that they have every right to lead a decent life. The second group doesn't."

Dr. Peretz defines that second group as "people who for a lifetime have had a special relationship to pain: looking for it, expecting it in varying degrees, anticipating it. So when it comes, to those people, it's no surprise. It's what they've been looking for. We're talking about people who hear that they've got a life-threatening disease and just give up. In a way, they welcome it. 'Come, sweet death.' They have always been afraid that something terrible was going to happen to them, and their way of dealing with the fear is to welcome it — to wait for it, and, when it comes, to embrace it. That's the undercurrent. It may not manifest itself that way. They may go through the motions of getting help, but they never manifest any real determination to get better, to live."

Whatever its source, whatever its strength, "Why me?" is a voice that every patient has to answer in his or her own way. Harold Taylor had the mental self-discipline to "abandon it, reject it, and keep it at bay" because "it would serve no purpose at all" and was "hurtful to [his] chances." Phyllis Kerr's feisty spirit relished the contrariness of being upbeat in the midst of so much pessimism and despair. Another patient I spoke to, who was told twenty years ago that breast cancer would kill her within six months, rejected "all that nonsense like self-doubt and 'Why me?' and 'I'm not good enough.'" She blames the media for spreading "the lie that life is a sitcom, or should be. In fact, everybody goes through illness. Disease is a part of life, an integral part. But we're not brought up to believe that. The result is that we tend to crumble in a crisis." Recently, the same woman had an operation for lung cancer. "To me, it really wasn't something to be taken too seriously," she says. "My ward lay directly underneath the pediatric ward, a ward full of babies with leukemia. I mean, in that context, how can you take losing a piece of your lung seriously."

That is a common refrain among the patients I spoke to. Whenever they begin to hear the inner voice of self-pity, the "Why me?" or "Poor me!" they think how much worse off they could be — how much worse off others are. "I try not to look at the 'Why me?'" says Gary Shields, the college student who fought testicular cancer, "because, as far as I'm concerned, I've been very fortunate. I've been blessed." Another patient with two small children used to pass the children's cancer ward every time she went to Memorial Sloan-Kettering for her own cancer treatments. "I would start to pity myself, and then I would walk into the lobby and see those kids there with no hair and IVs and amputations, and I would say to myself, 'And *you're* complaining?'"

Dr. Morton Silberman, the medical administrator turned patient, insists that throughout his ordeal with emphysema, he "never had a negative outlook," never once asked "Why me?" How did he do it? By telling himself, "There are things I can control and things I can't control," he remembers, and by thinking back to his boyhood on a farm. "I think my farming background helped me more than anything," he says. "Because as a farmer you learn that you can kill yourself quickly worrying about the things you can't control. You can't control the sunlight, you can't control the rain, and if you spend time worrying about the sun and the rain, you've wasted your damn time."

One time, however, like Phyllis Kerr, he felt his rural stoicism come close to cracking. It was in the early 1990s and he was "sick as hell." Of his many long stays in the Emory hospital (his hospital), this was the longest. "I had been in there a long time, and I don't know if I was getting depressed, or what," he recalls, "but that was the only time in my life that I really started feeling sorry for myself. You know, 'Pity me,' that kind of thing. And just about that time one of the nurses came into my room and said, 'Dr. Silberman, can I just stay in here for a while? I'm just coming apart.' She closed the door and sat there and cried for about an hour."

When she finally calmed down, she told Silberman what was wrong. "Have you seen this young girl walking up and down the hall?" Silberman recalls her saying. "She's a very pretty young girl about eighteen years old, a beautiful young girl." Silberman had, indeed, seen the girl. "Well, we took that little girl down for her scans today," said the nurse, "and, Dr. Silverman, she has cancer in her bones and in her lymph nodes, and she's not going to live another month. It just seems so horrible. You know, you see so much, and finally it just overwhelms you."

Silberman never heard the voice whispering "Why me?" again. "Here was this child who hadn't even learned what it's like to get out and live," he says, "and she was going to die. And I was still living. I thought, 'What the hell am I doing getting into a funk?' You don't have to look very far when you start feeling sorry for yourself to find somebody who's in much worse shape — and not just medically. Maybe they don't have any money, or, even worse, maybe they don't have any friends. Can you imagine: no support at all! Maybe they don't have people praying for them like I did. So how in the hell can you get down?"

What about me? How did I answer the voice that asked, "Why me?" in a hundred different ways every time I walked down the street, the voice that hounded me still as we circled over the forested hills of Virginia on the eve of surgery? My answer was this: I had been very lucky in my life, lucky in the broadest sense. Lucky with my family, lucky with opportunities, lucky with friends, lucky with talents. That luck (combined with some effort) had brought me a multitude of good things, an effusion of favors: a wonderful family, terrific friends, a fellowship in Europe, a

Harvard Law School education, a rewarding career, and a Pulitzer Prize, to name just a few. And *not once* in all those forty years of favors had I asked, "Why me?" *Not once* had I demanded of the universe a justification for those favors: a proof that they made some kind of sense. I had no right to turn around now and demand a logic or "fairness" for the bad in my life that I had never demanded for the good.

And this is what I told myself yet again, one last time, as the plane landed in Charlottesville.

My parents were waiting there for me; they had come on a separate flight (Steve and my sister would arrive the next day, the day before surgery). I was happy to see them, of course. They had brought me safely through many battles like this one. But the sight of their anxious, careworn faces brought me face-to-face with the one enemy that I had yet to master: guilt.

Guilt is perhaps the most unexpected enemy a patient like me has to fight. Often, it's guilt over putting family and friends through a wringer of anxiety and emotional turmoil. That's what it was for Gary Shields. "It really bothered me to watch my parents suffer," says Shields. "They were suffering more than I was suffering. Watching them worry about their child and knowing you're responsible is a terrible experience." But it can also be guilt over something as simple as leaving a spouse to carry on the burdens of everyday living alone and unassisted. It can be guilt over financial hardship, lost time on the job, lost opportunities for advancement, or just simply lost time. The burdens that life-threatening illness inevitably place on a patient's spouse and family don't have to be weighty in order to weigh heavily on a patient's conscience. I talked to one patient with a spinal cord tumor who was accompanied by her whole family from their rural home in the West to New York City for an operation. "I laid awake every night in the hospital," she told me, "worrying that they would get mugged, and I felt guilty for putting them in that kind of jeopardy."

215

Children are especially vulnerable to feelings of guilt — children of all ages. One doctor told me the story of an eight-year-old girl who, after she and her parents were informed of her advanced bone cancer, took her doctor aside and said, "I'm worried for Mommy and Daddy, because now they're going to be sad, because something bad is going to happen to me." "I think that there is a lot of guilt on the part of the child for putting their family through this," says Dr. Philip Pizzo, the NIH expert on pediatric cancer. "Parents often try to suppress their sense of anger and their sense of frustration, really suppress it deep down, but kids have extremely sensitive antennae for feelings like that, especially their parents' feelings. They pick up the signals and they feel that somehow it's their fault that Mommy and Daddy are upset."

Sometimes, the guilt that patients feel comes from an even higher source than parents. Dr. Richard Anderson, the oculoplastic surgeon at the University of Utah, remembers a seventy-year-old man who came to see him in 1976 when he was chief of the plastics division at the University of Iowa. The man suffered from blepharospasm, a rare disease that causes the muscles around the eyes to squeeze uncontrollably and severely, so severely that the eyelids stay shut and cannot be pried open. Like a lot of victims of blepharospasm, the man was essentially blind.

What was the treatment? "Until thirty years ago," says Anderson, "there wasn't any. Because of the strange facial contortions they made, people with advanced blepharospasm were usually dismissed as insane and often committed to asylums for life. That was the only 'treatment.'" In the 1960s, some doctors had limited success with removing the facial nerves, but it wasn't until the 1970s that a real "cure" was devised. And the doctor who devised it was Richard Anderson. By taking the squeezing muscles out of the eyelids, he made it possible for patients to keep their eyes open. "So people who had been functionally blind and considered crazy for years," says Anderson, "could finally find help." Anderson's operation has since been widely adopted as the preferred surgical treatment for blepharospasm, and it still bears his name: the Anderson myectomy.

The old man who came to him in 1976 was one of the first patients on whom Anderson tried his new procedure. The man was brought to him in a wheelchair. He had been functionally blind for twenty years. And for all those years, his family and neighbors had considered him crazy. Worse than crazy, in fact: *cursed*. "As is true with blepharospasm in general," says Anderson, "a lot of times people superstitiously relate the beginning of their blepharospasm to some other event." In this case, the other event was adultery. Twenty years before, this poor Iowa farmer had had an affair "in the corn field with the neighbor lady," Anderson learned, "and both he and his wife felt his strange condition was divine retribution for this two-decade-old indiscretion." Furthermore, they believed "that it couldn't be treated or couldn't be cured, basically because God was punishing him for his misdeeds."

But Anderson did cure him. "We did this extensive operation, removing all the squeezing muscles around his eyes, and for as long as I remained in Iowa, about ten years, he did well. He was able to keep his eyes open and see. From functionally blind in both eyes to seeing. He was one of the most grateful patients I've ever had."

Dr. Gordon Schwartz, the breast cancer surgeon, told me about "the saddest patient" he ever had. "She was a young woman who had been brought up in a strict Catholic home," he recalls. "She had never undressed in front of anybody. She had never gone to a doctor because she was embarrassed to get undressed." Left untreated for so long, her cancer had exploded. "She had cancer practically growing out her ears," says Schwartz. "And it was sad because she was the kind of person who thought she must have done something wrong and that God was punishing her for it."

Whether it was God's punishment, or just the long delay in seeking treatment, she died soon thereafter.

I didn't think I had done anything wrong, but God certainly seemed to be punishing my family. My parents had already lost one child. The day of my surgery, in fact, would be the twenty-first anniversary of my older brother's death in a freak climbing accident in California. He was twenty-one when he fell, and two decades later, my parents still visited his gravesite every Sunday after church. Since Bob's death, I had been my parents' only son. Now, as we drove from the airport to the hospital in the stone silence of small talk, I could feel them watching me, struggling with all the same old unanswerable questions. I could hear their special agony beneath the layers and layers of nonchalance in their voices, and I could see the painful memory of another death in their averted eyes. And all because of me.

And *that,* on the eve of surgery, was my greatest pain.

SIXTEEN

The Black Zone

ONE OF THE many ironies of medical problems like mine is that the hardest moment for the doctors and the worst moment for family and friends is often the easiest moment for the patient. That's the moment when you're out: when the rubber mask goes over your nose and mouth; the sounds of metal, glass, and porcelain fade; you lose track of the hands and faces and shapes moving all around you; and the lights of the operating room blur into the black zone.

Perhaps due to the aftereffects of the surgery, even the day before the operation remains something of a gray blur. The one memory that penetrates the fog of that long day is my first sight of Dr. Vinko Dolenc. We had talked many times on the phone and I had been impressed with his candor, his confidence, and his calm, reassuring voice, but I wasn't prepared for the tall, broadshouldered, commanding presence that strode into my room that morning. Later, I heard my sister, Linda, compare him to a 1940s matinee idol — of the wavy-haired, aquiline-nosed, suave, continental variety — but he seemed more American than that to me, despite his heavily accented (although perfect) English. He had a galvanizing optimism that seemed quintessentially Yankee — a can-do confidence that cast a brighter light in my room even than the Virginia sunshine flooding in the window.

Later that day, when they rolled me down to radiology for the inevitable angiogram and embolization preceding surgery, I needed all the confidence I could get, reflected or otherwise. Dr. Dolenc had laughed when I told him I feared these familiar procedures more than the surgery itself. But it was true. The fiasco at Mayo, and The Clamp, as well as the many long, torturous hours on the table in Dr. Hilal's grotto, were still painfully fresh in my memory.

After explaining my long history of bad experiences and my fears to the radiologist, I gritted my teeth and braced myself, waiting for the first whirring of the injection pump that would signal the start of another ordeal by fire. Only it never came. The pump whirred and sputtered, all right, but what came out was a new, noniodine, nonburning dye. That, and the constant ministrations of the radiologist, an extraordinarily skilled and sensitive man, transformed what I expected to be three hours of hell into merely three hours of motionless tedium. That night, the night before surgery, I sat in bed almost giddy with relief. As far as I was concerned, the worst was over.

Dr. Dolenc came by one last time to radiate another high dose of confidence. He also told me that, with my permission, he would be videotaping the operation the next day as a teaching tool, and if I wanted a copy of the tape, he would be glad to make one for me. A *videotape?* I thought. Hell, the only good thing about this operation was that I couldn't see it; that I wouldn't be around for it. The last thing I wanted to do was watch it on tape: not now, not a week from now, not ever. What was I going to do, show it to my friends? "Hey, everybody, grab a beer, take a seat, and let's watch my brain surgery!"

All I said was "No, thanks."

Early the next morning, after a surprisingly easy night's sleep, they came to take me away. I had risen even earlier to shower and shave (as if I were going out on a date). From my first waking moment, I felt different than I had ever felt before on a morning like this, different than before the big surgery in Los Angeles, certainly; but different even than before the experimental procedures in New York. I felt it even as they rolled me down the endless series of halls and elevators that led to the OR, a feeling so new that at first I didn't recognize it. Indeed, it wasn't until my very last minute of consciousness, when I felt the rubber mask on my face, that I finally was able to put a name on it.

Optimism. After years of feeling panic in every unguarded moment, after years of grim prognoses, dire scenarios, and just plain fear; now, in the most unguarded moment of all, the only feeling in my fading awareness was a buoyant, beaming optimism.

What gave me that feeling, of course, was knowing that I had done everything I could — pursued every option, interviewed every doctor, weighed every decision — and that all that effort had led me inexorably to the right place, at the right time, with the right doctor — this place, this time, this doctor.

And a good thing, too. It was certainly too late to turn back.

I closed my eyes and slept the dreamless sleep for twelve hours.

SEVENTEEN

All the Difference

DR. WILLIAM BLAISDELL, the senior trauma surgeon at the University of California at Davis, wasn't supposed to be flying into the Sacramento airport on that Sunday evening in December 1993. He was supposed to be at a conference in Chicago. But when the conference was canceled at the last minute, he and his wife decided to come home early. She was in the seat next to him, the window seat. Just after the plane began its final approach, she looked out the window and saw a cluster of flashing lights on the edge of a country road. "Uh oh, dear," she said to her husband, "I think there's an accident down there." After spending so many years with a man who made his living putting people back together after accidents, she felt uniquely "attuned" to scenes like the one below. Her husband, on the other hand, didn't even bother to lean over and look. "I thought nothing of it," he recalls.

Until he got home, that is.

The phone was ringing when he walked in the door. "Did you hear that Bobby Hurley was in an accident?" It was the team physician for the Golden State Warriors. The Warriors were scheduled to play the Seattle Kings, and reports of a car accident involving the Kings' star player were all over the news. The great Bobby Hurley, multimillion-dollar athlete extraordinaire, "King of the Kings," was near death.

Blaisdell immediately called his hospital. "Yes," the doctor on duty told him, "Hurley is here. We're just taking him to the operating room. I believe he's ruptured his left main bronchus. *Can you come in right away?*"

The bronchi are the tubes that connect the main airway, the trachea, to the lungs. Each is about the diameter of a thumb. When one of them is torn away from the lung completely, it is usually, according to Blaisdell, "an instantly fatal thing." In all his years of doing trauma surgery, he had never seen a ruptured bronchus in a patient who was still alive.

But Bobby Hurley was alive — although, when he heard the story of his accident, Blaisdell didn't know how.

After finishing a game, Hurley had left the stadium and was driving along a remote road not far from the Sacramento airport. As he crossed an unlit intersection, a car with no lights on came hurtling out of the darkness and slammed into the side of Hurley's open Jeep. Without his seat belt buckled, Hurley shot out of the open car like a rocket — reporters later measured his "flight" at more than a hundred feet — and landed in a watery ditch at the side of the road. The force of the impact crushed his left shoulder, pushing it deep into his chest cavity; shattered his left leg, deranging his knee; and tore a deep gash down his left side, exposing muscle all along its path. And his head was underwater.

That's where Bobby Hurley's bad luck ended — and his good luck began.

He was lucky that someone happened to be out walking a dog not far away, saw the accident, and pulled him from the water before he drowned. He was lucky that one of his teammates was following not far behind, saw the accident, and called 911 on his car phone. Lucky because it was a slow Sunday night for medical emergencies and the ambulance arrived within five minutes. Lucky because the accident happened almost in the shadow of U.C. Davis Medical Center, home to one of the best trauma centers in the country. Lucky because the chief resident there had just finished writing a chapter for a book on trauma that Dr. Blaisdell was editing — a chapter on a very unusual kind of injury: tracheal bronchus ruptures.

Another doctor might not have recognized that the sinking in Hurley's chest every time he took in a breath was a sign of severe damage in one lung. Another doctor might not have known that when they put him on a ventilator and he "blew up like the Michelin tire man," it meant that this standard treatment for trauma patients would kill him in a matter of minutes. Another doctor might not have known that the regular breathing tube should be replaced with a special divided tube that allowed one lung to be ventilated but not the other, injured lung. "That was the key to immediate survival," says Blaisdell. "With a ruptured bronchus like that, you cannot use assisted ventilation because the air leaks out through the hole."

But most of all, Hurley was lucky that Dr. Blaisdell wasn't in Chicago that night. Working straight through till morning with a team of other surgeons, Blaisdell found the ruptured bronchus — it had, indeed, been ripped completely loose, leaving the left lung "hanging by its blood vessels." At that point, another doctor might have just taken out the lifeless lung. Indeed, most doctors would have. "Under most circumstances, in the average patient," says Blaisdell, "I would not have chanced his life, but would have taken out the lung. But I weighed the odds: If I took out his lung, there was no going back. If I left it in and we had a complication that was life-threatening, he was such a good physical specimen that we had a margin of safety in which he could tolerate a major complication."

So, in a long and delicate procedure, Blaisdell sewed the lung and bronchus back together. For the next three days, the breathing machine dutifully pumped air in and out of the injured lung. On the fourth day — "the critical time," according to Blaisdell — they removed Hurley from the breathing tube and held their own breath. After a few halting tries, he started breathing on his own — with both lungs.

Unfortunately, not every patient is as lucky as Bobby Hurley. Many people live far from major trauma centers like Blaisdell's, and one-third of America isn't covered by 911 emergency service at all. "If you have a severe injury and you can stay alive and get to an acute care center within half an hour," says Dr. Richard Marder, the orthopedic trauma surgeon who repaired Bobby Hurley's knee, "then you have a chance. But if Hurley's accident had occured in any one of a number of places in this country instead of where it did, he simply wouldn't have made it." Another doctor who worked on Hurley called his injuries "ninety-eight percent fatal in the field."

For Bobby Hurley, luck made all the difference.

Fortunately, however, most patients don't need luck — they don't have to be "in the right place at the right time," or live close to a major medical center, or have the right doctor on duty when they're brought in. Most patients with a life-threatening medical problem, like me, have the one thing Bobby Hurley and other trauma patients don't have: time. With enough time, any patient can *make* his or her own luck. With enough time, any patient can go out and investigate various therapies, find the best facilities, pick the best doctors. With enough time, any patient can prepare — mentally and physically — for the ordeal of treatment and recovery. And for most patients, it's this combination of the right doctor, the right treatment, and the right attitude — not luck — that makes all the difference.

It's what made all the difference for Carol Ohnemus. She was fifty when she started having trouble breathing. But it wasn't until she took a new puppy out for a walk and had to struggle to keep up, that she knew it was time to see a doctor. Not that the doctor was much help. He gave her an antibiotic, and when that didn't work, gave her a different antibiotic. Meanwhile, it just got harder and harder to breathe. Then the emergencies began. Over the next eight months, she was rushed to the hospital four times with "pulmonary emboli," blood clots in her lungs. Her blood clotted so rapidly that they started referring to her around the hospital as "Clotty Carol." But they still didn't know why.

Then, in January 1993, on a trip to Kansas City, her lungs shut down altogether. She reached the hospital in time, but after that, "things went downhill in a hurry," she says. They sent her home on oxygen and she stayed on oxygen the rest of the year. Only she needed more and more oxygen. "I could only be up and about for an hour a day," Ohnemus recalls. "And even that just wiped me out." By the end of the year, she was confined to a wheelchair. "I felt like I was dying," she says.

And still the doctors weren't any help.

She tried specialist after specialist. One said he couldn't do anything for her because he had to test her blood, but to do that he first had to take her off blood thinners, and she was in such bad shape, he was afraid if he did that she would "throw some more clots." Another one agreed that clots were the problem but he couldn't tell where they were, which meant he didn't know if he could operate. Another one said she would have to lose weight before he could operate — "but how can I lose weight when I can't exercise because I can't breathe?" she asked. Another one suggested putting her in the ICU and "just experimenting with different kinds of drugs to see what would happen."

While the specialists debated, her condition worsened. She had to leave the door open and the fan on when she took a shower because the humidity made it so much harder to breathe. The "big effort" of every day was unloading the dishwasher. Simply lifting her hand above her head caused her to break out in a sweat.

And all the doctors could do was confirm and put numbers on the harsh reality she was living every day: Her pulmonary artery was 95 percent blocked by clots. Her breathing capacity was 48 percent. Her life expectancy was six months.

Then she found Dr. Nicholas Kouchoukos, the cardiothoracic surgeon at the Jewish Hospital in St. Louis — the right doctor with the right treatment: surgical removal of all the blood clots in her lungs and pulmonary artery. "Clotty Carol" provided the third ingredient. "This was a woman who wouldn't take no for an answer," Kouchoukos recalls. The result was, by the reckoning of both doctor and patient, a miracle. After the operation, Ohnemus considered it a miracle that she woke up at all — "Just the mere fact that I knew I was alive."

For Kouchoukos, the miracle was in Ohnemus's recovery. Over the next months, her breathing capacity went from 48 percent to 84 percent; she left the wheelchair and oxygen behind. "We don't resurrect too many people from the dead," says Kouchoukos, "but this lady was one of them."

Another patient for whom the right doctor, the right treatment, and the right attitude made all the difference was Charles Adkins, an oil company employee in Houston, Texas. Adkins was fifty-three in 1983 when his family doctor found a strange lump in his abdomen. It was the first time he had ever had anything wrong with him. "Cancer was one of those things that happened to other people," he recalls, "it didn't happen to me." Only this time, it did. Adkins was diagnosed with renal carcinoma, cancer of the kidney — "big as your fist," he brags, Texas style, "the largest ever in the history of Baylor College of Medicine."

Adkins and his wife, Doris, were surprised and scared, but they "didn't fall apart," according to Doris Adkins. Only a year before the diagnosis, they had lost their eighteen-year-old son in an automobile accident, and Doris, for one, was determined she wasn't going to lose another member of her family. Unfortunately, the first doctor they consulted mistook their determination for denial. On the day that Adkins was scheduled for surgery, he told Doris that neither she nor her husband were "taking this illness very seriously." "Don't you realize," he told Adkins in his wife's presence, "that you have a ninety percent chance of *not* surviving this operation?"

Furious, Doris Adkins backed the doctor against the wall. "We *are* serious about this," she said, "and we *are* worried. My husband does *not* want to lose his life at this point, and I certainly do *not* want to lose my husband. I've had enough loss for one lifetime."

But words were not enough. With her husband literally on the way to the operating room, with the blood to his kidney already cut off in preparation for the procedure, Doris stopped everything. "Something inside of me just triggered," she recalls. "I'm not usually a belligerent person, but it's different when I'm protecting my family."

"This is not going to happen," she told the startled doctor. "I had to lose one member of my family without any hope. And you've just tried to kill what little hope we have here, and that is not satisfactory. I'm not going to accept it."

"Well, I'll have you know I'm considered the second-best doctor in this field in this area," the doctor sputtered.

To which Doris Adkins replied acidly, "Well then, why don't you just use your clout and get me the best one."

And that's how she found Dr. Peter Scardino: the right doctor with the right treatment. Scardino was able to remove the entire tumor, and because it hadn't metastasized, Adkins did not require either radiation or chemotherapy. Seven years later, he had another tumor, this one "as big as a baseball," he says, also malignant, in the same cavity between his aorta and intestine. Scardino removed that one, too. In the thirteen years since he was first diagnosed, Adkins has seen his daughter graduate from college and marry and now he's a grandfather. "And at one time I didn't know whether I'd see any of that," he muses. "That's my idea of a miracle."

Indeed, on Dr. Scardino's staff, Adkins is still known as "the walking miracle."

Every doctor has stories like Bobby Hurley or Carol Ohnemus or Charles Adkins, stories of people for whom the right treatment, the right doctor, and the right attitude made all the difference — whether it was the difference between breathing and not breathing, walking and not walking, or life and death. Dr. Martin Malawer, Tamara Enoch's surgeon, has saved countless limbs, preserving not just "whole" bodies, but the "whole" lives that go with them. Dr. Joel Cooper, Ann Harrison's doctor, has done the same with lung transplants. "This is certainly a field in which, if patients don't find their way to one of the people doing cutting-edge work," says Cooper, "they can have a very different end to their stories."

Another transplant specialist, Dr. Michael Sorrell, told me about a woman in a small Arizona community who wasn't allowed into any of the stores in town because everyone thought she had leprosy. "It was like *Ben Hur*," says Sorrell. "This woman was a pariah in her own community, an outcast." In fact, the woman had a rare liver disease that caused a buildup of cholesterol in her joints. At Sorrell's direction, she underwent a liver transplant and the ugly deposits "melted away." "She was like a new person," Sorrell recalls, "not only from the new liver but from a whole new outlook in life because she wasn't this outcast any longer."

An absolute cure, of course, isn't always possible — even with the right doctor, the right treatment, and the right attitude. Sometimes "the difference" is measured in less dramatic terms: the length of recovery, the severity of side effects, the amount of pain, the freedom of movement, the frequency of complications. But there are also times when the difference is *more* dramatic than merely cure or no cure. There are times, in fact, when the difference is between cure and catastrophe. Dr. William Wood, the cancer surgeon, told me about an emphysema patient, not a smoker, who complained of shortness of breath and blackouts. A major medical center told him that bronchial plugs in his right lung were choking him during the night and therefore that lung would have to be taken out. The man was prepared to have the operation until, at the last minute, his son-in-law, a doctor, flew into town and forced him to get another opinion. "I had him seen by a series of people," recalls the son-in-law, who was Dr. William Wood, "and they did find the things described, but none of them really believed that it was a tight explanation. They weren't happy with it, and they were concerned that if this right lung was taken out in a person with severe emphysema, he would really be a pulmonary cripple. He wouldn't be able to do anything."

So Wood kept looking until he found a doctor who recognized his father-in-law's real problem: an extremely rare condition involving spasms of the vocal cords caused by mucous plugs from the bronchial tubes hitting the larynx. The doctor gave him a slant board and a few simple procedures to reduce the plugs and told him to take a Valium at bedtime for a few months to help him relax. *And that was it.* He never had another problem. "And to think he could have had a lung taken out unnecessarily," says Wood, "and been a cripple the rest of his life. He probably wouldn't be alive today, which he is. He would have lost a lung, and for what? Nothing."

And what was *my* difference? How did the combination of the right doctor, the right treatment, and the right attitude work for me? Well, to start with, I woke up. Like Carol Ohnemus, I considered just being alive the first and most important miracle. Only five years before, I might never have emerged from that dreamless slumber. Even better, I could *feel* the nurse touching my wrist and ankle for a pulse, I could *hear* the regular beep of the heart monitor, and, once they gave me some ice chips, I could even *talk* — although for a long time the effort required was more than I could muster.

Another difference: I could see. Out of both eyes — although when someone approached my bed from the right, I saw two figures instead of one. I knew who I was (that was the first question they asked me when I blinked awake, "What's your name?"). That one was easy. The tough ones — like whether and how much my memory had been affected, would come later — although, even in my groggy state, I wondered how I would know if I had forgotten something. Had I simply forgotten the name of my third-grade teacher or had it been cut out of me? Neither, in fact. Mrs. Davis was her name. Phyllis Davis. I would close my eyes and test myself like that for hours in the bustling solitude of the recovery room, running through the huge library of my life looking for missing pages.

The second time I blinked awake, I was surrounded by faces. And I recognized them all.

EIGHTEEN

Angels

WHEN PHYLLIS FORBES KERR woke up after her longest and most dangerous surgery, the first person she saw when she opened her eyes was her mother. "She was standing over me," Kerr recalls, "and I swear to God she looked like she had a halo around her head."

My mother was the first person I saw, too, when I woke up in the recovery room after surgery. Then my father, my sister, and Steve, all standing around the bed, *all* looking like they had halos around their heads. (With all due respect to Kerr, I think it had something to do with the bright overhead lights in the recovery room and my eyes' sensitivity to the glare.)

Every patient needs an angel, whether it's a mother, father, sibling, spouse, or friend. Every patient needs an angel like Louise Enoch. "I had to keep myself together for my daughter," says Louise. "I was the only parent she had. An eight-year-old like Tamara can only understand so much." (The same can be said about patients of every age.) During her daughter's long hospitalization, Louise never lied to her, never hid anything from her, and let her help make all the decisions. During the even longer recovery, Louise continued both to comfort and to exhort. When Tamara lost all her beautiful long blond hair to chemotherapy, Louise made a game of wigs and costumes. But when she balked at resuming school, Louise made her go. "I wasn't going to let her sit at home and wallow in self-pity," she says.

Every patient needs an angel like Melissa Taylor, who accompanied her husband, Harold, to every interview with every doctor across two continents "because I was convinced that people can perform their best if they feel someone is going to appreciate it and if someone is there to nudge them along." When her husband ran into problems with hospital bureaucracy, however, Melissa could do a lot more than just nudge. "We hit some bumps along the way," she recalls, "and immediately I went straight to the hospital administrator. Because I think whatever experience you are passing through, if you have an opportunity to make something better for a person that is close to you, you must."

The experts all agree: Every patient needs support — not just during recovery from an operation like mine, but all during the long course of catastrophic illness, from diagnosis to (one hopes) cure. Support is the final ingredient — after the right doctor, the right treatment, and the right attitude — for making medical miracles happen. "Educating yourself to choose the right course of therapy and the right physician, having a will to live, and having a support network, those are the big three," agrees Dr. James Kirklin, the heart surgeon, "but it's the last of those that's the strongest." According to Dr. Andrew von Eschenbach, the urologic oncologist, research has shown "that prostate cancer patients who have support over and above their therapy do better than those who don't. This phenomenon has been apparent to physicians for a long time. What none of us has understood are the underlying mechanisms."

Some of those "mechanisms" are not so hard to figure out.

With a major illness, where survival is at issue, especially one like mine that drags on over months or even years, people wear out; they get exhausted. "Having patients fully involved is a good thing," says Dr. Dorothy White, the pulmonary specialist at Sloan-Kettering, "but I have found over the years that patients occasionally need the rest and peace that come from somebody taking care of them. That's where both their doctor and their support network can help."

Support can instill the will to live where it doesn't exist, or strengthen it where it does. "In the majority of cases," says Dr. Robert Rigolosi, a prominent nephrologist at Holy Name Hospital in Teaneck, New Jersey, "the support of the family is probably the most important factor in the will to live. I've seen cases where if it hadn't been for the family, the patient would not have gotten the same attention. Where everybody, all the doctors, the nurses, *and* the patient were ready to throw in the towel, but the family wouldn't let them. No doubt about it: There are patients who would have been dead if they were alone."

Dr. Kirklin observes that support is particularly important for patients who have a low sense of self-worth. "There are a lot of people who don't consider themselves special," says Kirklin. "And when a physician tells them that there is nothing more to do, they are likely to say, okay, there is nothing more to do." For people like that, it's often the support network, whether it's family or friends, that introduces fight into the equation of survival. "They're the ones who say, 'I want everything done, dammit.'"

According to the NIH's Dr. Philip Pizzo, that kind of support can have a beneficial effect all its own, not only on a patient's illness, but even on his or her life. Pizzo cites the case of an inner-city African American girl with an "incurable" soft-tissue tumor whose family was told, "Take her home, nothing can be done for her." The girl's aunt, however, refused to give up the fight, and with the help of Candlelighters, an advocacy group for children with cancer, found Dr. Pizzo, who put the girl on a course of experimental chemotherapy that has kept her alive for the last fourteen years. (She recently graduated from law school.) "It's easy to measure the favorable impact of a drug on a disease," says Pizzo, "much harder to quantify the favorable impact of the kind of support that girl received."

The patients I spoke to didn't understand the "mechanism" of support any better than their doctors, but they certainly understood its effects. Luana Cruz was twenty-six when she woke up in a hospital bed with rods in her legs. The last thing she could remember was driving home from her waitressing job. She didn't remember the accident or the thirty hours of surgery in which doctors tried to save her legs — "They didn't know if I would walk again," she recalls, "but they were sure I could never waitress again." When they asked about her family, Luana told them she didn't have one. In fact, she did, but she hadn't seen any of them in more than a decade. ("It was one of those adolescent things that got out of hand," she admits.)

But Luana did have an angel. "I had my boyfriend to support me," she recalls. "He was basically my only support at the time, the only person who stood with me through this whole thing. And he was there for me one hundred percent, every day. Most guys probably would have taken off. But he stuck it out and didn't give up on me." Joan Teckman, the swimmer with cystic fibrosis, had two angels who stayed with her for two months after her transplant operation while she learned to breathe with her two new lungs. "My sisters came in every day and told me, 'Oh, you're so pink,' and, 'Oh, you look great,' and I kept looking at them saying, 'You're lying to me.' I kept thinking that I was really doing very, very poorly, and no one was being honest with me. But they just kept coming in and kissing me and saying, 'You look great.'" Teckman speaks for legions of patients when she says of her two angels: "They're the whole reason I'm alive."

That kind of support comes in every shape and style. It can be as simple and easy as a hospital visit or as complicated and onerous as an organ donation. For Darren Weber, the soldier whose parachute failed to open, the mere fact that his family — all eight of them — flew to his bedside was support enough. "We're not a real huggy, huggy family," he confesses, "so I didn't really expect it. But when it counted, they came through. That meant a lot." Another patient's eighty-seven-year-old mother took a more "military" approach to her support. "She would come into my hospital room like a drill sergeant," her daughter remembers. "She had me moving and out. She would say, 'Okay, now get up. I want you to *walk*.' She's that kind of person. She never gave up and she never gave in." A schoolteacher-patient woke up from her mastectomy operation to find that her students had hung a huge Marx Brothers poster in her room, "so I would laugh when I woke up every morning," she recalls. When Phyllis Kerr was undergoing the agony of radiation treatments, she and another patient would leave notes for each other underneath a chair cushion in the waiting room. "I so looked forward to those notes," she says. "They really lightened the burden."

One thing is for sure: Whether it's Louise Enoch's fierce maternalism or Melissa Taylor's patient partnership; whether it's Doris Adkins lambasting the doctors for their pessimism and snatching her husband out of the OR or Luana Cruz's boyfriend simply *being there* at her bedside every time she woke up; whether it's Phyllis Kerr's beatific mother or Joan Teckman's effusive sisters; whether it's Carol Ohnemus's father and husband standing quietly at her bedside or Bobby Hurley's endless parade of basketball dignitaries extolling his courage to the media; whether it's posters on the wall or notes under the chair cushion, support is support is support, and everybody needs it. "You really do need all the help you can get," one oncologist told me. "This *is* that rainy day you're always talking about."

For Jacquelyn Mayer Townsend, that rainy day came only seven years after Bert Parks crowned her "Miss America for 1963." She was twenty-eight, married, the mother of two beautiful children, and still beautiful herself. In short, she had a lot to be thankful for on that Thanksgiving day in 1970 — despite the severe headache she had all day long. The next morning, she woke up to the sound of her nine-month-old daughter, Kelly, crying for her bottle. But when Townsend started to get out of bed, she couldn't move. She tried to raise her head, but couldn't. She tried to sit up, but couldn't. She tried to lift her arm, but couldn't. She tried to lift her leg, but couldn't. Nothing on the right side of her body would move. Kelly's cries went unanswered. And soon they were joined by her mother's cries.

Townsend woke her husband, John, to tell him something was horribly wrong. But she couldn't speak. She moved her mouth, but no words came out. All she could do was cry. And she did lots and lots of that. "I was terrified," she recalls. "I didn't know what was wrong. I was like a prisoner in my own body."

At the hospital, they determined that she had had a stroke — probably an adverse reaction to the birth control pills she was taking. When people talk about life-threatening illnesses, they don't usually mention stroke — not among twenty-eight-year-olds, at least. But stroke is one of the major causes of death and disability in America. As Jacquelyn Townsend learned. Within hours, she was lying in the intensive care unit of the local hospital, paralyzed in more ways than one. "I really did not know whether I would live or die," she recalls, "and I tried to stay awake the whole time because I had this feeling that if I fell asleep, I wouldn't wake up."

Before long, however, friends and family began to gather. Her husband and children, her own family from Ohio, her husband's family, all appeared outside her ICU door, and one-by-one, for brief periods only, filed past her bedside. She couldn't talk to them. She had to communicate in writing, on a tablet, scribbling awkwardly with her left hand, or just pointing to words already scribbled. Every day, John would take her for a walk down the hospital corridor, dragging her right foot behind her, a little further each day. Sixteen days after she arrived, she left the hospital and went home in a wheelchair.

That's when Jackie Townsend's angels appeared. And they came in the form of children. First, her daughter, Kelly, helped her learn to talk again. "She was nine months old, and she and I learned how to talk together," Townsend recalls, "which was wonderful, because we competed with each other. If she could talk better than I could, then I would really work harder to talk better than she could."

When she could talk again, Townsend's five-year-old son, Billy, took over as teacher. "He had learned his ABCs in school," Townsend recalls, "and I couldn't remember how my ABCs went. But if Billy said 'A,' then I could say 'A' after him. I had also forgotten how to count, so he helped me with that, too." Her husband was supportive, of course, says Townsend, despite a job managing a racetrack that kept him away from the house days and sometimes nights. "But Billy was my real teacher because we were together every day after he came back from kindergarten."

He taught her how to tie her shoes again, how to make the knot in her belt or the bow in her scarf. "The child became the mother to the parent," Townsend recalls. "Things I had taught him, he had to teach me." As she progressed to cooking again, Billy would read the directions and she would follow them. "I can remember we made a cake once, and instead of putting baking powder in the cake, I put baking soda in it, and of course the cake didn't rise. But he let me make my own mistakes. 'That way you'll learn from them,' he told me. He was a good teacher." Of course, he would laugh whenever "Mommy did silly things," but they always laughed together. "The laughter was wonderful," says Townsend. "It made everything a lot easier to bear. More than anything else, Billy taught me that I shouldn't be so serious about overcoming. You work hard, sure, but you have to laugh sometimes."

Jackie Townsend knows how lucky she's been. Today, twenty-six years after her paralyzing stroke, she walks and talks with a hint of her former disabilities that only she notices. "I still hesitate when I'm speaking," she says, without any sign of hesitation, "especially when I'm tired." But she never seems to tire. She carries on an active schedule of speaking on behalf of stroke victims, advocating prevention, detection, and prompt treatment. "The most important thing to remember," she says, "is that a stroke is an emergency, so get to a hospital right away."

Like so many patients, Townsend takes no credit for her remarkable recovery. The credit, she insists, belongs to "my two little angels," both of whom are adults now. She also worries about patients who don't have the support she had. "If the family runs away or is not there to support and encourage," says Townsend, "then the stroke survivor, or anyone who is disabled, really doesn't *want* to come back. Some do, but I've found that if you don't have anyone there to encourage you, you just don't improve. So it's really the family, the friends, the people that the stroke survivor comes in contact with, who have to be understanding and care."

Like Jackie Townsend, I was one of the lucky ones. From the very beginning of my long ordeal, I was never without angels. At my very first hospitalization in Cambridge, friends from law school, and especially from the Harvard Glee Club, made my bedside a busy place. Years later, when I rushed to Mayo at Christmastime, one of those Glee Club friends, Rick Kvam, was a student at Mayo Medical School. Rick was always preternaturally wise and calm, even in his "wild" college days; and that wisdom and calm brought light and air into the darkest, most claustrophobic week of my life.

I agree with Jackie Townsend (and Norman Cousins) that laughter is a powerful tonic, and during my first major surgery in California, I was lucky enough to share the companionship of the funniest woman on the planet, Sarah Fitzsimmons, who worked on the PBS series I was writing (and who later went on to write for the TV show "L.A. Law"). Within weeks of the surgery, when my head was still wrapped in a huge bandage that made me look like a giant Q-Tip, Sarah insisted that I accompany her on her anthropological expeditions through the mall culture of Southern California, and made me laugh so hard I was sure my stitches would pop.

And then, in all those places, and everyplace in between, there was Steve.

When people talk about support, they tend to think in terms of responding to a crisis. It's an image deeply fixed in our culture: flying to the hospital bedside of a loved one, flowers or candy in hand, offering soothing words, encouraging blandishments, vicarious fortitude, whatever. Such a selfless, ennobling drama. In a society that largely suppresses public displays of emotion except in the most formalized and circumscribed ways ("You may kiss the bride"), a hospital visit is an opportunity to show one's sentimental side in full sail.

But that's only part of the story — the part they show on daytime soaps. Most patients need support — need it more, probably — long before the admitting nurse clips that little plastic bracelet on, long before the flowers and visitors start arriving. Especially in cases of protracted illness, like mine, the need for support can stretch over months, years, or even decades. That's why every patient needs a Steve. From the big decisions about doctors and options, to the minutiae of renting an apartment (and towels and dishes) in a faraway city where I could recover from surgery, Steve was there. From the morning my consonants disappeared to the day I could whistle again — and felt like doing it — Steve was there.

But if Rick, Sarah, and Steve were all my angels — and they were — the archangel, without doubt, was my mother.

It is curious how often mothers come up when I talk to other patients about their ordeals. And not just Louise Enoch. Gary Shields, the college student with testicular cancer, sounds the common theme: "My mother is a very strong person," he says, "and she wasn't about to give up. She sat there in that hospital room for *two and a half years*."

Of course, my father and sister came for the operations, too; but it was my mother who stayed. It was my mother who nursed me back to health after the first brain surgery in Los Angeles. I can still remember the look on her face the first time she saw me without that giant Q-Tip bandage: my swollen, discolored head and great, crescent-shaped wound. I could see her wrestling to subdue the great surge of maternal sympathy, the horror and the revulsion, all at once. Until finally, "It's looking better," she said brightly (like Joan Teckman's sisters, "You look just great").

And now, ten years later, it was my mother who moved into the little apartment off Rio Road in Charlottesville that Steve had found and, with only a few pieces of rented furniture and a load or two of necessities from the local Kmart, somehow managed to make a "home" for me to recover in. I don't know whether it was just her daily presence after so many years of my being on my own, or my return to the infancy of infirmity, but it was as though thirty years had suddenly dropped off my life. I was ten again, in bed, home sick from school. Mom was in the kitchen making me soup. Jackie Townsend and her kids had a reversal of roles; Mom and I had a reversion.

Not all was sweetness and sepia-toned light, however. To be fair, I was not an easy patient. The post-op medications I was on, mostly steroids, made me short-tempered and moody and demanding in ways I instantly regretted. In addition, the peculiar nature of my surgery and the location of the tumor made me hear and see things that didn't exist. It was not an agreeable combination. "Turn off that radio," I would shout from my bed to my mother in the kitchen — when, of course, there was no radio playing. Partly, too, I was frustrated by the glacial pace of healing.

Every day, we took walks around the apartment complex, measuring my progress in numbers of steps or circumambulations of the building. The double vision increasingly worried me. I couldn't drive, couldn't read, certainly couldn't write. Would it go away? Dr. Dolenc seemed convinced that it would. The eye specialist was more guarded. Between them, the uncertainty made me anxious and testy — literally: Every day, I tested my vision (as I tested my memory) to see if there had been any change.

And partly, of course, it was the guilt.

Fortunately, both my mother and I knew from our previous ordeals together what too many patients are surprised to discover: Catastrophic medical problems, like mine or Jackie Townsend's, are hard on both patients *and* those who support them. Being an angel is hard. At times, downright hellish. Inevitably, patients are at their most vulnerable: ashamed of the way they look because of chemo, radiation, or scarring; and distracted by the rebellion in their bodies — from the illness or the treatment or both — nausea, headaches, diarrhea, disorientation. For all these reasons, plus the often unpredictable effects of medications like steroids, they can act like different people altogether: irritable, dismissive, abrupt, forgetful, thoughtless, selfish, childish (the list is depressingly long). Even total personality changes are not unknown. One neurosurgeon told me about a patient who, after brain surgery, wanted to give up his lucrative legal practice and move to the South Sea Islands. "I feel like a new person," he told the doctor as he planned his getaway.

When Dr. Robert Brumback, the trauma surgeon, has a patient with "devastating injuries," he makes a point of sitting down with the family and explaining, "Listen, he's going to be okay. He's going to make it. He's going to live. But *he's never going to be the same.*" Brumback describes what experience has taught him is the usual "arc" of recovery. "He's going to get mad at you, he's going to throw things, he's going to call you names, and he's going to be depressed. But you can't make this any better, and that's going to be very frustrating for you. That phase may take six weeks or six months or six years, but you'll know when it's over. And it *will* get over. You're just going to have to ride it out, because that's all you can do."

Brumback identifies the two most common reactions to serious illness, among both patients and their supporters: anger and depression. But while friends and family can take it out elsewhere, patients usually take it out on the people closest to them — just as I did. Diane Blum, the executive director of Cancer Care, warns patients about "the tremendous strain that a diagnosis of cancer puts on a family: the emotional stress, the physical stress, the financial stress. Even family relationships that were solid beforehand," says Blum, "can deteriorate because of cancer." Dr. Pizzo at NIH often sees parents fighting over their sick children. "There is no child or family that goes through a catastrophic disease unchanged," says Pizzo. "Nobody stays neutral. They either change for the better, which absolutely can happen, or the whole organic structure of the family can fall apart." All too often, it's the latter. "I often see parents of children with brain tumors split up," one neurosurgeon told me, "which is very sad, but it doesn't surprise me."

Virginia Andriola, who directs a brain tumor support group, has seen families come apart at every seam: siblings angry at siblings, parents at children, children at parents. "Illness just destroys families," Andriola laments, "any kind of illness, but especially chronic illness. An episodic illness, you can band together and get through it. A chronic illness — whether it's a brain-injured child or a disabled spouse — a chronic illness doesn't affect one person, it affects the whole family. It affects each person in the family differently, but it's tough on everybody."

And toughest of all on spouses.

Life-threatening illness is hard on relationships in general, but for all the same reasons, it is hardest on marriages. Andriola tells the story of a woman in her thirties whose husband had had brain

surgery to remove a tumor "and just never was the same again."
The woman not only had to care for her disabled husband, she
had to assume full responsibility for their eight-year-old son. Five
years later, when her husband's tumor recurred, the woman filed
for a divorce. "She just couldn't take any more," Andriola says.
"She stayed with him for five years. That was as much as she could
take. And it's hard to blame her. She had no life. She had no marriage. Sexually, he wasn't there for her, and she had all the responsibility. Now here he was, dying, and she would have had to take
care of him even more."

"You'd be *amazed* how many marriages break up after brain
surgery," says Columbia-Presbyterian's Bennett Stein. Dr. Stein's
assistant, Pat Farrell, who has been an angel herself to legions
of Stein's patients (including me), sees firsthand how marriages
come apart under the strain of major surgery. "Sometimes the
spouse who doesn't have the tumor is angry at the spouse for having the tumor," says Farrell. "They are angry at the world. Sometimes it's the person who has the tumor. They're angry at the
world, too. And they take it out on their spouse."

Farrell attributes the high rate of breakups first to drugs.
"Ninety-nine percent of the patients are put on steroids after
surgery," she says, "but often their families are not made aware of
the side effects — the irritability, the personality changes. They
can go into depression, they can get paranoid, they can get high
as a kite, they can start eating like there's no tomorrow, or they
can lose their appetite. Some people think they're going crazy.
And it's all strictly from the medicine, and people are not aware
of that."

But, Farrell admits, there is an emotional element, too. "When
a person with a life-threatening problem gets through the surgery,
often they are like a new person, and the person they've been living with all these years can't deal with that new person." The
lawyer who wanted to quit his legal practice and run away to the
South Seas (literally, not figuratively) didn't have any intention of

taking his wife of twenty-five years with him. Farrell advised the wife to "just bear with it. He'll get over it." She did, and he did, and they both backed away from divorce. "But they're the exception," says Farrell, "not the rule."

Both Stein and Farrell have also noticed that many marriages seem to get through the anxiety of the preoperative wait and the rigors of the surgery itself, only to come unglued afterward, during recovery. "Both the patient and the family can be wonderful when they're going through the surgery," says Farrell, "they really hold up. And then, two or three weeks down the road, they fall apart." Dr. Stein has a name for it: the brink-of-death syndrome. "As long as they're focused on getting through the ordeal, they're fine," Farrell explains, "but then when everything is going to be okay and the pressure is off, they suddenly realize, 'I could have died!' *Then* they go crazy."

And they're not the only ones. Ann Harrison reports that the same is true of lung transplant patients. "The number of marriages that break up either just before, during, or after transplant is horrendous," she says. "They're dropping like flies." *Before* the transplant, it's usually the supportive spouse who wants to bail out, according to Harrison. She tells the story of a patient who went home and told his wife that he was going to have a transplant. "I don't think you should do it," was her response, "and if you go through with it, I'm leaving you." He was stunned, but had the operation anyway. And she did leave him. Harrison doesn't know if she left "because she couldn't handle the idea that he was going to be healthy, or because she just didn't want to go through the ordeal." The husband, who is "doing great," doesn't know either. "The wife has called him a few times, and she'd like to get back with him," says Harrison, "but he won't have anything to do with her now. He says, 'She couldn't stick around when I needed her. Now I don't need her, and I don't want her.'"

When the breakup comes *after* the transplant, on the other hand, it's usually the patient who wants to jump ship. "Sometimes it's just pure selfishness on the transplant patient's part," says Harrison. "They want to be free" — like the lawyer with dreams of escaping to Tahiti. Harrison has known women who were "totally dependent on their husbands before their transplants, then afterward "let their hair grow long, put makeup on, go on drastic diets, start wearing miniskirts, and all this. They want to get out, they want to *live*. Off with the old, on with the new."

But, in fact, it's the men who are more likely to feel this postoperative wanderlust, according to Harrison. "Men find it really hard to be sick," she says, "so when they get back on their feet, they want to go, go, go. In general, the women just deal with it better than the men." By way of explanation, Harrison suggests that because transplant programs don't accept patients over a certain age, many of the men undergoing the operation are in their prime midlife-crisis years. The medical crisis doesn't create new problems, it just brings existing ones to the surface.

And *that* is the key, according to the experts; that is the reason so many relationships are weakened or wrecked by life-threatening illness. It's tempting to think that a medical crisis turns *everybody* into an angel. It's practically a cliché: Somebody is diagnosed with a frightful illness and everybody rushes to the bedside. Problems that loomed large the day before suddenly seem trivial, old animosities are buried, family rifts are healed, old slights forgiven. Everybody rallies to meet this new, unexpected, overshadowing, life-and-death challenge.

Unfortunately, it doesn't always work that way. "Both patients and their supporters expect each other to act differently as a result of a serious illness," says Virginia Andriola, "kinder, gentler, whatever; when, in fact, you can't expect someone's personality to change just because they're sick — or just because you're sick."

Suzanne Post found that out the hard way. In 1985, after a long bout of fatigue and troubled breathing, she was diagnosed with emphysema. The doctors told her "nothing could be done at all," she remembers. "I was just going to be on oxygen for the rest of my life and that was it, end of story." Well, not quite. Using her contacts at the state university, where her husband was vice chancellor, Post started networking and researching and ended up in the offices of (who else?) Dr. Joel Cooper, as a candidate for a high-risk, double lung transplant.

Because she had done her homework, Post was prepared for the long, roller-coaster wait for an appropriate donor (she was wheeled into the operating room five times only to be sent back when they found something wrong with the donor lungs). She was prepared for the Homeric ordeal of recovery: the physical and emotional pain, the degradation (carrying oxygen everywhere she went), and the embarrassment (when one of her sons was married, she had to have oxygen waiting for her at the front of the church). What she wasn't prepared for — the "biggest surprise of all," she calls it — "was how people acted." Not the strangers who wondered what was going on: "They were kinder than anybody," she says. No, she is talking about "friends, even family. The people you think would be the most sympathetic and the most helpful — I mean, you need a ton of help — you never see them at all. You scare them to death. They just want to run away. They just hope that you don't die while they're in the room with you. I couldn't believe it. Some members of my family acted like absolute mental patients, really. It truly stunned me. I always thought if you got critically ill, everybody would be sympathetic and rush to your aid. But it's just not true."

In fact, life-threatening illness by itself doesn't turn anybody, patient or supporter, into an angel. It doesn't transform people. If anything, it only makes them more like themselves. Far from smoothing over or resolving problems — in people, in relationships — it tends to *magnify* them. Whether it's a friendship, a marriage bond, or a family tie, any relationship that is already weak is only more likely to fray under the strain of catastrophic illness. "Nobody gets sick in a vacuum," says Andriola. "And those preexisting personality and family structures don't change. If anything, they get more rigid and inflexible *because* of the illness. However a couple communicated before in times of stress is exactly how they will communicate, or not communicate, in times of illness. If a husband is impatient with his wife's moods, he's not going to be able to cope when she has a breast removed. People bring to bear on a medical crisis all of the strengths *and* weaknesses that they had prior to the crisis."

Dr. Robert Brumback, the trauma surgeon, tells of "obnoxious, unfeeling people whose personality faults are magnified by their accidents and their bad behavior is now accepted because of their condition. It's frightening sometimes to see how much their spouses have to put up with. The accident gives the injured person more power: 'I need this' and 'You are going to get this for me.' Life-threatening illness magnifies all family problems like that."

What do patients do when they're not one of the lucky ones; when, unlike Jackie Townsend or me, they don't have angels in their lives; or when, like Suzanne Post, their would-be angels "just want to run away and hope that you don't die while they're in the room"; or when, as in Ann Harrison's case, they "can't handle the idea that you're going to be healthy," or just "don't want to go through the ordeal"? Robert Knutzen, the president of a support group for patients with pituitary tumors, says simply: "I sit and cry for the ones who have no support."

But Suzanne Post was not the kind to sit and bewail her fate. She knew she couldn't count on her busy husband — "You can only push people so far," she says. "A lot of patients want the spouse to be there for them twenty-four hours a day, but that wasn't going to happen, and there was no point in trying to make it happen." Her kids lived in different, distant places. They called a lot, but basically their lives were centered elsewhere, so they couldn't be much support, either. "But that was probably okay," says Post. "I don't know how much they could have stood up under the pressure. In a way, the closer the person is, the more difficult it is for them. Besides, you shouldn't expect one person in your life to rush to your side and want to stay there forever and give up his or her own life. They're not going to do it, and you'd both be sorry if they did. As a patient, I realized that I couldn't impose that burden on one person, anyway. I had to spread it around a bit. So I just rounded up as many other supports as I could."

In fact, that is exactly what the experts recommend to patients who, for whatever reasons, find themselves without angels. "One of the most important interventions we make," says Cancer Care's Diane Blum, "is to try and help people broaden their network of support." In many cases, Cancer Care itself becomes a part of that broadened network. It provides free counseling, education, and even financial assistance to anyone with cancer, their family members, and friends. "That's exactly what we're all about," says Blum, "trying to support individuals and families through an illness that for most people is the most difficult thing they've ever experienced in their lives."

Cancer Care, and many organizations like it, work with patients to see "who else in their lives can be supportive of them," says Blum. "Do they have friends? Do they have other family members? Is there someone at work? You must be realistic about the stress that being diagnosed and being treated puts on you. This is a time when you really do need all the help you can get."

For many of the patients I spoke to, that help came from their doctors. For Joan Teckman, the swimmer with cystic fibrosis — as for many lung transplant patients — the angel in her recovery was Dr. Joel Cooper. "Some doctors are so busy with the scientific aspects of what they do," says Teckman, "that they can't accommodate the emotional side of a patient's needs." But not Dr. Cooper, who called every night during Teckman's recovery, "to see how I was doing and if I needed anything."

Gary Shields felt the same way about Dr. Donald Skinner. Shields, like Suzanne Post, found himself alone sometimes, even in a crowd of concerned family. His fifteen-year-old brother was too devastated himself to cope. His older sister was married with a life of her own on the other side of the country. His parents were strong and supportive but conflicted about the rightness of the experimental procedure he had chosen. It was Dr. Skinner who "pulled the family together," says Shields. "He was so compassionate, and so positive, and so optimistic that we had made the right choice — that everything was going to be fine and that there *was* hope. Because of him, it all came together."

For some patients, nurses can still be the "angels in white" of popular imagination and historical fact. But the changing nature of nursing is making that role harder and harder. As Pat Farrell points out, "Nurses are working two or three days a week, twelve hours a day now. So if you become attached to one in particular, they are with you a couple of days but then they're gone for a week. And by the time they come back, you're probably out of the hospital." That's one of the reasons Farrell finds herself increasingly walking the wards of the Neurological Institute, stopping to talk with Dr. Stein's patients and their families, "even though that's really not part of my job. I go see the patients, and they ask me questions, and it makes them feel that somebody cares."

Some patients look to other patients for support. Tamara Enoch is still best friends with a girl she visited in the hospital before her surgery. "She had lost her leg," says Tamara, "but she hadn't lost her spirit. She was a great influence on me, on everyone." "The advantages of being able to talk to somebody who has had their own personal experience with the same problem can't be overestimated," says Andrea Hecht, head of the Cushing's Tumor Society. Like most of those active in patient support groups, Hecht was a patient herself once. At age twenty-two, she was diagnosed with Cushing's tumor, a deep-brain pituitary tumor, and it was only after ten years of missteps and costly lessons in becoming an aggressive patient that she found the right doctor and the right treatment. "A doctor can't look a patient in the eye and say, 'I understand where you've been,'" says Hecht. "That's why I tell doctors, 'You take care of the patients' physical needs, let us help take care of their emotional needs.'"

Many of the former patients I spoke to eagerly make themselves available to other patients — patients who are just beginning their ordeals, patients who are caught in a lonely, familiar place. Jackie Townsend speaks out on behalf of stroke victims. Ann Harrison is nothing less than a legend among lung transplant patients and still tries to meet every single transplant candidate who comes into the hospital in Toronto where she had her operation. "They really want to see somebody who's been done," she says. "And I walk in and say, 'Hi, my name is Ann Harrison, and I've been transplanted for ten years.' And they just say, 'Oh, my God, you look so great. I can't believe you had a transplant. Just seeing you is half the battle.'" Richard Bloch, founder of the H&R Block tax consulting business, who survived his own harrowing ordeal with lung cancer, has written a book about it, and still spends much of his time, through his family's cancer foundation, fighting the fear and ignorance that continue to surround and obscure this devastating disease. "It's so rewarding," he says of his cancer work. "We get such gorgeous letters from people. It's so much better than making money."

In short, there are angels everywhere, and they come in every guise. Not just as mothers or fathers or husbands or wives or small children reciting their ABCs. They come as nurses and doctors, as fellow patients, as friends and co-workers, as support groups, as 800 numbers, even as total strangers. What makes an angel an angel — what "gives them their wings," as Jackie Townsend puts it — is the needs they meet: for the patient, the need to be cared about; for the supporter, the need to care. And, ultimately, it's hard to say which is the greater need. For, as my mother reminded me every time I apologized for "all the trouble" when she guided me around the block for the hundredth time or dressed my ugly wound and told me yet again how much better it looked: "Not to be loved is tragic," she said. "But not to love is catastrophic."

NINETEEN

Embraced by Life

WHEN DR. ROBERT BRUMBACK, the trauma surgeon, tells a patient's family that their loved one "is going to be OK *but he's never going to be the same person again,*" the patient isn't usually present. Indeed, the patient is usually still unconscious in the recovery room. Yet, Brumback admits, the person who most needs to hear that message, the person who invariably has the hardest time accepting it, isn't a member of the family. It's the patient himself. "There's a part of the problem that all the family support in the world, important as it is, can't solve," says Brumback. "Ultimately, the patient has to deal with it himself."

Just when a patient thinks he's passed the final test, scaled the final mountain, survived the final trial of catastrophic illness, comes the biggest challenge of all: living with the consequences. "The most interesting thing to me about the patients that I have," says Brumback, "is their denial with regard to what their life will be when they're done. The hardest pill to swallow — and I wish there *were* a pill for it — is the realization that from the moment the accident or illness or operation occurs, your life will never be the same. Everybody assumes that they're going to be back to the way they were. They're going to be in the same job, they're going to have the same physical capabilities. Their work, their spouse, their family, their friends, everything is always going to be the same. When, in fact, it will never be the same after."

After?

Like a lot of patients, I never thought about "after." I was too wound up in "before." It wasn't denial so much as desperation. And priorities. Who can think about the future when there's so much going on in the present? The life-and-death decisions are all in the present; the obstacles, the challenges, the dangers, all in the now — or at least in the soon. It was everything I could do to figure out a way to *have* a future. ("Just let me see my fortieth birthday," I used to whisper to myself late at night.) Who had time to worry about what happened then? To think about after was to think about *not* after — the possibility that there wouldn't be an after.

So, like a lot of patients, I wasn't prepared for after.

But it is absolutely true, as Brumback points out, that no patient comes through a medical catastrophe unchanged — whether it's the sudden and traumatic kind of catastrophe he deals with, or the long, drawn-out kind I was dealing with; a car accident or cancer. And those changes can have a profound, often unexpected effect not only on a patient's relationships, but also on the patient.

Some patients, of course, are lucky. They come through even the most horrific ordeals with their lives only slightly altered. Darren Weber limps a little. Tamara Enoch can't wear shorts. Jackie Townsend has some numbness on one side of her face and her memory isn't as good as it used to be (whose is?). Fortunately, I was one of these. Except for the usual huge scar and bald pate, both of which would disappear with time, the only life-altering change I had to face was the double vision in my right eye.

I use the word "only" here retrospectively, out of admiration for patients like Weber, Enoch, and Townsend, and what they had to overcome. At the time, however, it didn't seem like "only." Even three weeks after surgery, I still couldn't drive, couldn't read, and most disturbing of all, couldn't write. The eye doctor at U.V.A. gave me a pair of special lenses that were supposed to eliminate the ghost images that haunted my right field of vision, but the only thing they brought into focus was a headache. The only way I could do anything, even watch TV, was to close my right eye, and I quickly became adept at keeping it closed for long periods of time (throughout a movie, for example). But that, too, gave me a fierce headache. In general, I dealt with this change in my life with a combination of denial and hope — denial that it was really so bad, and hope that Dr. Dolenc, not the eye doctor, was right; that it, too, would disappear with time and, yes, my life *would* be the same again.

Even when my mother returned from the pharmacy with an eye patch, I still refused to swallow Dr. Brumback's "pill of realization" that my life, in fact, would *never* be the same.

Imagine, then, how much harder it is for patients who are not as "lucky" as I was, whose lives have suffered profound and permanent changes as a result of their ordeals, to swallow that pill. Dr. Brumback tells of a highly skilled construction worker whose catastrophic injuries required amputating both legs. "The machinery he ran was not set up to run with all-hand controls," Brumback recalls, "and the company wasn't about to take the risk and go to the expense of putting that guy back on the job. No way. Yet he had been doing that job for twenty-five years, so he just assumed he would eventually go back to it." According to Brumback, "We're not set up as a culture, or maybe as a species, to accept the fact that once my leg is amputated, I need to adjust things in my life. That adjustment is very hard. Losing a limb is losing your self-image of what you are in society."

In one form or another, every patient faces the problem of adjusting to "life after." For an example far more common and closer to home, one only has to look as far as the nearest smoker.

The denial that makes it possible for a double-amputee construction worker to "just assume" he will go back to his old job running heavy equipment (or, indeed, for a half-blind writer to just assume he will go back to writing), is exactly the same denial that makes it possible for a double-lung transplant patient to light up a cigarette.

"It really is stunning," says thoracic surgeon Nicholas Kouchoukos, "how many patients go back to smoking after a lung operation or back to drinking after a kidney operation. They may stop for a while, but as soon as they begin to feel better, they put the operation out of their minds and drift back into it." Dr. Edward Rosenow, chairman of the Division of Thoracic Diseases at the Mayo Clinic, tells his AIDS patients, "Each puff is shortening your life span. Your quality of life can be better and I can help you with your AIDS, but you must quit smoking because it's *killing* you." But still they smoke. Another doctor warns his patients, "If you keep smoking, you *will* get lung cancer. And you only have a one-in-ten chance of surviving lung cancer." And still they smoke.

One frustrated surgeon told a lung-transplant patient that if he caught her smoking, "he would reach down and take her new lungs back." (In Canada, a patient *has* to quit smoking to be eligible for a heart-bypass operation, and a lung transplant patient who resumes smoking can't get a second transplant.) Another thoracic surgeon told me that he once found a lung cancer patient of his lying on the bathroom floor in her hospital room, dead, with a cigarette in her hand. "A patient who refuses to take care of herself not only compromises her recovery," says Kouchoukos, "but inevitably has an impact on her doctor's motivation to help her. You have to take responsibility for your own life."

And *that* is the point.

Every doctor I spoke to agreed that, at some point, a patient has to take responsibility for his or her own recovery. "Ultimately," says Dr. Rosenow, "your life is in your control." Not smoking after a lung transplant operation is only the most obvious and dramatic example of the kind of "adjustment to life after" that patients have to make. Every patient has to adjust to new limitations. One young patient at Columbia-Presbyterian was so eager to recover his former life, that as soon as he left the hospital after brain surgery, he "walked to all the places he and his girlfriend used to walk," his doctor recalls, "the museums, the park, down Madision Avenue." The effort so exhausted him that he spent the next six months despondent "over his lost vigor and, he thought, his lost life." In contrast, another neurosurgery patient decided to "gauge" her activity after leaving the hospital. "I knew if I went out and had fun one night," she told me, "the next day I would pay for it. The pain would be really bad. It was just a fact of life and I learned to budget myself."

For a lot of patients, pain is the most difficult adjustment to life after: whether it's "budgeting" pain, managing pain, avoiding pain, or learning to live with pain. Here again, I was one of the lucky ones. The headaches that hit like an earthquake every time I tried to read the paper, and rumbled through every TV show, and rocked me to sleep every night for weeks after the surgery, gradually began to subside. But for many patients, pain and its management become part of their new, post-illness identity. Just as some patients refuse to come to terms with limitations on their activities, some expect to return to the perfect, pain-free world of their previous lives. "A lot of my patients have been in pain for a long time," says Dr. Brumback, "and they lean on things like narcotics a lot. Crutches like that can be just another way of refusing to accept that catastrophic illness changes your life forever."

Ultimately, the truest measure of a full and successful recovery isn't how little pain a patient has to endure, or how much of their energy returns, or how many working limbs they have — or how well their eyes work — or how noticeable their limp is, or their scar, or the slur in their voice. The truest measure of a full recovery is whether a patient successfully responds to the changes that catastrophic illness brings into their life; whether they deal with the inevitable "adjustments," from trivial to tectonic, that those changes demand; whether they cling to their old life through anger and denial, or embrace their new one — and are, in turn, embraced by it. "Some people have the mental outlook to handle even the most horrible injuries," says Dr. Brumback. "They say, 'I can live with this. I'm lucky I'm alive.' Other people are just devastated. They never, ever make the leap to being a constructive human being again."

When doctors told Phyllis Forbes Kerr, at age twenty-four, that because of her cancer she could never bear children, she was despondent at first. "Then I realized this was a great chance to adopt," Kerr recalls. After that, she focused her energies on the battle with adoption agencies who didn't believe she would live long enough to raise a child — a battle that she ultimately won. Thirty years later, her son is grown and the child every mother would want to have. "Cancer didn't deprive us of having children," says Kerr. "In fact, we feel our son is particularly special because of everything that happened."

Ann Harrison survived one of the first double lung transplants just fine, but weeks later when her rehabilitation nurse brought her to the top of a flight of steps, she thought her life was over. "I'd never been so scared," she recalls. "I hadn't used stairs in ten years. It must be what a child goes through when they first contemplate going down a flight of steps." Like a child, Harrison was embarking on a new life, a changed life. For her, unlike most patients, the change meant a return to "normalcy" — but a normalcy as unfamiliar, frightening, and life-altering as life without a limb. "You take so long to get sick," says Harrison, "then suddenly you have to adjust to life with lungs."

After the marathon thirty-hour operation to save her legs, Luana Cruz looked at the pins in her legs and listened to the doctors telling her all the things she would never do again — like make her living as a waitress — and told herself, "I've got the rest of my life. I can't just dwell on what has happened." Whenever during the long recovery she felt her strength fade or she grew impatient over her slow progress or the pain threatened to overwhelm her — "pain like I'd never felt before; having a baby was nothing compared to this pain" — she remembers telling herself, "Nobody can make you better, you've got to do it yourself. I mean, the doctors can only fix you so much, and if you don't do the rest, then . . . ," she leaves the sentence unfinished.

Luana Cruz's "life after" required one last adjustment: She reunited with the family she hadn't seen in sixteen years.

No one ever embraced life after catastrophic illness with more courage or determination than Sean Lavery. When Dr. Brumback describes with admiration how some patients "make the leap" from devastating injuries to "being a constructive human being again," he must have Sean Lavery in mind.

Certainly, no one's life changed more.

Lavery was twenty-eight when he first noticed a tingling in his leg — "like cold water running down my calf," he recalls. To anybody else, it wouldn't have seemed like much — just one of those strange, inexplicable aches and pains that accompany everyday living. But Lavery wasn't just anybody. He was a dancer. And not just any dancer. He was a principal dancer with the New York City Ballet, one of the premier ballet companies in the world.

Even so, Lavery ignored it at first. "I just thought my back was out of whack," he recalls. He was a dancer, after all, and dancers have those kinds of problems — "kinks" — all the time. They push their bodies hard and sometimes their bodies complain. Nothing unusual in that. Then, a year and a half later, in the middle of a performance, he noticed that his left foot was "acting strange." It wouldn't point right. It didn't give him a solid take-off for his spectacular jetés. "It just wouldn't obey me," he says.

Still, Lavery brushed it off. He was just tired. It was the end of a long season. And, indeed, after the season ended and he could take some time off, it didn't bother him again. Until the next season. As soon as he started exercising to get in shape for the West Coast tour that opened the new season, he noticed that his left leg had atrophied. He attributed it to some surgery that had been done on that knee six years before. It just meant he would have to redouble his efforts to strengthen that leg before the tour began.

But the leg got worse, not better. He could still dance. Indeed, on tour, he danced two ballets a night, "but I felt like I was dying," he remembers. "I couldn't hold up my left side. Everything was more difficult than it should have been." But still, he told himself he was just out of shape. "I thought, 'Oh, God, I'm old at thirty.'"

Then, on the opening night of the company's 1986 season in New York, in the middle of his dramatic pas de deux with the ballet's prima ballerina, Patricia McBride, it happened. "I was just walking to the corner of the stage," Lavery recalls, "nothing fancy. I took a step with my left foot, and suddenly I couldn't feel where my foot was. I knew right then: Something was definitely wrong."

After seeing a series of doctors, he found out just how wrong. At thirty, Sean Lavery was diagnosed with a spinal cord tumor.

Not long after that, Lavery was sitting in an office that I knew well: the office of Dr. Bennett Stein at Columbia-Presbyterian's Neurological Institute. After looking at Lavery's scans, Stein told the young dancer, "I can't promise you anything. I can't say, 'Oh, you'll be fine.' All I can say for sure is that you have a spinal cord tumor. We won't know exactly what we're dealing with until we get in there." When Lavery asked what were his chances of *dancing* again, Stein told him, "fifty-fifty." Later, Stein revised those odds to "thirty-seventy."

On the eve of surgery, Sean Lavery, like me, wasn't thinking about "after." "I was thinking about my *life*," he remembers. "I was thinking, 'Oh, God, what if it's malignant?' The career was of course a concern, but the more immediate issue was whether I was going to live or die."

The surgery lasted eight hours. When Lavery regained consciousness in the recovery room, he made a devastating discovery. "My left leg was paralyzed," he recalls. "I couldn't move it at all. That answered any questions I had about my career. It ended right there." A dancing career that had begun when Lavery was a ten-year-old boy in Harrisburg, Pennsylvania; a career that had drawn him at the age of thirteen to New York City, where he lived with his ballet teachers; a career that had seen him turn professional at sixteen and join the New York City Ballet at twenty; a career that had attracted the approving eye of George Balanchine himself (it was Balanchine who gave Lavery his first principal role when he was only twenty); a career every dancer wishes for but few have, was effectively ended. Like Dr. Brumback's construction-worker amputee, Sean Lavery was without the only work — the only identity — he had ever known.

Two days later, he started therapy.

Lavery was already losing the battle against self-pity when the orderly came to his bedside for the first time, wrestled him into a wheelchair, and rolled him to the physical therapy room, where another orderly wrestled his upper body into a harness, planted his feet on a mat, then hoisted him onto his limp leg. There was a time when his pirouettes on that leg were a thing of beauty. Now he was an ungainly marionette in excruciating pain. "That first day I felt pathetic," he recalls.

But his attitude quickly changed when he started to look around and see the other patients in physical therapy. "Some people were just trying to sit up without falling over. They had big scars on their heads, obviously from brain tumors. I looked around and I thought, 'I'm really lucky.' I don't want to sound like a Pollyanna, but when I saw what other people were going through, people who were dying up there and people who couldn't say their names, I thought, 'Oh God, am I lucky.' I mean they couldn't control their bowels, they were wetting themselves. I thought, '*Who cares if I never tendu again!*'"

But he did want to walk again. And before that, to stand up again. So twice a day, he endured the agony of the trip up to the physical therapy room. And the humiliation of having to call for help to go to the bathroom in the middle of the night. Then they had to reoperate to stop a leak of spinal fluid. "That was the worst pain I've ever felt in my life," says Lavery. When he learned to use a walker, they put a metal brace on his leg so he wouldn't stumble over his own limp toes. The *New York Times* came to do a story — "A Dancer's Nightmare" — but Lavery resented the camera. "I looked like Frankenstein," he says, "with this big metal brace on my leg. It looked like I had made it in shop class." After more than a decade of dazzling audiences all over the world with the beauty of his movement, Lavery was stumbling and camera-shy. A month after the surgery — as soon as he could stand up with the aid of the walker — he escaped the hospital ("Get me out of here!") and hid from the public eye.

But the hospital turned out to be a vacation compared to Marika, the ballet company's physical therapist. "She really whipped me into shape," Lavery recalls. "She took one look at that walker and said, 'Get rid of it.' She was very aggressive and she knew me, and she knew what dancers could do, the discipline they have." For four hours every evening, Lavery and Marika met at a friend's aerobics studio. "She would chase me around the room," Lavery recalls, "and do all these things with me, like teach me how to walk correctly, because I just couldn't."

There was a time there, Lavery admits, when he thought about dancing again. He didn't talk about it; he didn't even let himself think about it much, and then mostly in the middle of the night. "I was desperate to get back to the stage," he recalls. "At that point, that was all I had. I had been a dancer for twenty years, and here I was, at thirty, at the height of my career, and boom, it was over. So I was working my butt off to try and get back."

And the work was paying off. He *was* making remarkable progress. Everyone agreed about that. He was getting his feeling back much faster than anybody expected. By April, only four months after the surgery, he was off the walker and onto crutches. He spent exactly one day on crutches before jumping to a cane. "They were all flipping out at how fast I was recovering," he remembers, "or that I was recovering at all." When he started, nobody was sure if he would walk again. Now no one doubted he would walk, but they were still saying he would never dance again. Maybe they would turn out to be wrong about that, too. "You've made such progress," they would say, shrugging their shoulders. "Who knows?"

For Lavery, the moment of truth came when Marika pulled him into a studio, tossed a pair of ballet shoes at him and barked, "Okay, put these on. Let's go. Let's try ballet."

"Are you out of your mind?" Lavery replied. "I can't even walk right." But he knew what she was trying to do. She knew the fantasy he was harboring.

"Well, let's see," she challenged. "It may trigger something in your mind. It's something you've been telling your body to do for years. So if you can do it, you can do it."

That was Sean Lavery's last dance. "I knew immediately, this is not going to happen," he remembers. "I couldn't feel my leg. I still limped. I knew there was no way I was going to be doing jumps and complicated maneuvers when I didn't have complete feeling in my foot, in my whole leg. I realized then that even if I did get back to dancing, I wouldn't look as good as I did when I quit, and who needs to see that. It was time to get on with my life."

A year after his surgery, Lavery returned to the New York City Ballet — not to try and reclaim his former life, but to embrace a new one, as a teacher in the company class. He had made Dr. Brumback's "leap." And he still feels lucky. "I danced just about everything you could possibly dance," he says. "I joined a major company when I was twenty. I danced for Balanchine. I'd had it all. Sure, I could have been doing it longer. Sure, I would have preferred to decide the right time to retire. But it didn't happen that way. I danced great ballets, and I danced a lot. Not many people can say that."

After his first year teaching, Lavery was asked by the company's director, Peter Martins, to organize a benefit performance for the Dancer's Emergency Fund, which provides financial support to dancers, like Lavery, facing serious crises in their lives. Lavery not only organized the evening, he hosted it. When he walked out in front of the packed house, with a barely detectable limp, to make a speech on behalf of the Fund, the audience rose to its feet. "It was incredible," Lavery recalls. "I thought they'd just applaud politely, like 'Oh, yeah, we remember you.' But it was unbelievable. The applause just wouldn't stop."

TWENTY

"I'm Still Here!"

DR. JOEL COOPER, the transplant surgeon, tells the story of a patient who was transferred to M.G.H. in 1968 when he was chief resident there. She had severe respiratory problems, and her case history read like a textbook on complications: endless intubations, bleeding, and seven operations. When she finally limped off the ventilator six months later, Cooper used her as an example of a patient "it would have been easy to give up on. We were all a hundred percent certain that there was no chance that she could possibly survive, and yet here she was."

But, in fact, he didn't expect her to live long in that condition. "She had lung function which was terrible, and one horrendous, horrendous, impossible sort of problem after another, leaving her alive, but just barely."

In 1993, when he received a second round of media attention for the development of an operation for emphysema (the first round being for his first-ever successful lung transplant in 1983), Cooper got a card in the mail from Florida. "Dear Joel, I was so delighted to see that you're still performing miracles." It was from the same woman who had limped out of the hospital twenty-five years earlier. "I am alive and well and living in Florida with not too many problems for a sixty-nine-year-old woman."

It was signed "Still here, Shirley."

Dumbstruck, Cooper immediately called Shirley and arranged to see her on his next trip to Florida to visit his parents. "I couldn't believe it," he recalls of their breakfast together. "She was playing golf. She looked the picture of health. She had remarried. I was absolutely flabbergasted not only that she was alive, but that she was doing so well."

Every doctor has stories like Cooper's, stories of patients who won't give up, even when their doctors do; patients who persist long after others have stopped trying; patients who are, to everyone's amazement, "still here." "One of the few positive things about getting sick," says Alice Trillin, "is that people find out that they can do things that they never thought they could do."

Certainly, no one thought Betty Robinson could do what she did. Robinson was forty-eight and on her way to the dentist when a truck came out of nowhere and plowed into the side of her car. Fortunately, this wasn't one of those "big city accidents," as she called them, where ambulances come and people are rushed off to emergency rooms. After all, this was Coffeeville, Mississippi, a town of about five thousand halfway between Jackson and Memphis, Tennessee. After her head stopped rattling, Robinson went on to the dentist, then drove her limping car to the body shop. "I didn't think I was hurt," she recalls. "I thought I was lucky."

But just to be safe, she went to see her family doctor, who examined her, took some x-rays, and agreed: She was, indeed, lucky. All she had was a sprained ankle and a bruised shoulder. "He didn't think I had a serious problem," she recalls. Robinson wasn't surprised. By her own telling, she had "never been sick a day in my life — never even had a headache. I was the kind of person who opened my eyes in the morning, got up and out of bed, and was ready for the day."

When she opened her eyes the next morning, however, her neck was swollen, aching, and flaming red. She went to see a neuro-surgeon in Jackson, who had taken care of her daughter when she broke her neck in another car accident several years before, but he couldn't find anything. He gave her some therapy to do at home and told her to get as much bed rest as possible.

Two *years* later, she noticed her right foot was starting to drag when she walked. And her fingernails were numb. She went back to the neurosurgeon in Jackson. This time, he found something: Her top two vertebrae had separated and pulled away from her skull. One was pressing on her brain stem, the other on her spinal cord.

She needed an operation.

The neurosurgeon sent her to Birmingham, Alabama, for sur-gery because "he didn't operate on friends," Robinson recalls. She considers that the first of many missteps. "The surgeon in Birm-ingham had a bad, bad personality," she says. "He was real short with me and real rude." After the operation, when she started having earaches and ran a temperature of 104, he told her, "You don't have a problem," and accused her of being a hypo-chondriac — "Me, who never even had the flu!" Robinson drove home and told her husband. "That doctor doesn't want to have anything to do with me."

She lived with the pain for another year and a half, including six weeks of futile therapy in a Memphis hospital where the doctors told her, "There's no hope, Mrs. Robinson. Nothing can be done." Robinson was despondent. "My doctor in Birmingham didn't want me. My doctor in Jackson died of a heart attack. I didn't have anybody to go to." Finally, she resorted to another family friend, a doctor in Atlanta. What he saw shocked him. Now, in ad-dition to everything else, her reflexes had become spastic.

Even after a battery of tests and scans, he couldn't find what was wrong, but he referred her to a neurologist in Alexandria, Vir-ginia. Robinson and her husband drove to Virginia, only to be told, after another round of tests, that she had "pressure on the nervous system." "But," said the neurologist, "I don't know where it is, and I don't know what to do about it." Her "only hope," he said, was a special clinic in Switzerland. Later, out of Robinson's hearing, the doctor confided to her husband, "I wouldn't touch her with a ten-foot pole."

Next, she tried a spinal rehabilitation center in Birmingham. After six weeks of therapy there, they told her she "didn't have any more pressure," and sent her home.

Only, the symptoms didn't go away. Her leg was still dragging, she was still losing her balance, her face still burned, and her reflexes were still spastic. The only change was that now she had *another* symptom: Her eyes "jiggled." "They would track together fine as long as I was totally still," she recalls, "but if I moved at all, one eye would go one way and one would go another." Every time she took a step, she felt nauseous. "It was horrible."

She went to an eye specialist, but all he could tell her was, "Your eyes may never get any better, but they won't get any worse."

Robinson was at her wit's end. She told her husband, "I just don't know what to do."

But she kept looking. An old boyfriend of her daughter's who had become a surgeon directed her to yet another neurosurgeon, this one in Nashville. "Mrs. Robinson," he concluded after examining her and doing yet another set of scans, "you do have a problem."

"Thank you, Doctor," said Robinson flatly. "But I know that. Can you help me?"

"No," said the doctor, just as flatly, just like all the others, "there's nothing I can do for you." Also like the others, he gave her the name of yet another doctor, a specialist he had studied under in New York. "Do you mind traveling to New York?" he asked.

"I'll do anything," said Robinson. "I'll go anywhere."

The doctor in New York was Bennett Stein.

"I went in and met Dr. Stein," Robinson recalls. "He had my scans up on the board, and he looked me in the eye and said, 'Mrs. Robinson, I have good news and I have bad news. The bad news is you need surgery. Without surgery, you probably have six months to live. The good news is, with surgery, you have a sixty percent chance of coming through it and a forty percent chance of being totally paralyzed.'"

Three weeks later, Stein did the surgery. Robinson spent two months at Columbia-Presbyterian, flew home by ambulance jet for exactly one night — which she spent in the local hospital — then headed to Tupelo, Mississippi, for rehabilitation.

By the time she arrived, she was choking to death. The rod and bone fusion that had been done during her first orthopedic operation wasn't holding. Her chin was falling over on her chest, closing off her throat and making it hard to breathe and impossible to swallow. The doctors in Tupelo had to do an emergency tracheotomy with just a little Novocain, no anesthetic. "It was absolute agony," Robinson recalls.

In fact, her whole time in Tupelo was agony. "They were horrible to me," she remembers. "They would sit me up in a wheelchair and leave me for hours, and I couldn't hold up my chin, and it was beginning to cut off the oxygen to my brain." She couldn't raise her arms. She couldn't leverage herself out of bed. She couldn't turn over. Her teeth were locked together. She couldn't talk. She had to "eat" through a feeding tube. She couldn't swallow the saliva in her mouth and she couldn't raise her hand to wipe it away when it dribbled out. "It was a nightmare," Robinson remembers. "Here I am, this grown woman, who's really kind of a tough person, and I'd sit there with tears running down my cheeks in absolute agony."

When she left six weeks later, she told the doctor she was going to New York to see Dr. Stein again — "Maybe *he* can do something for me," she sputtered. The Tupelo doctor's response: "There is nothing that can be done for you, Mrs. Robinson, and they will never touch you again. And if they do anything else to you, I guarantee that you will be totally paralyzed."

She went to New York anyway.

Dr. Stein immediately put her in traction, flat on her back, spread-eagled, with a metal ring around her head and fourteen pounds of weight to pull her spine back in line and get her mouth to open. She lay like that for twelve days. At one point, one of her team of doctors came in and, seeing her ordeal, said, "Betty, you must come from good stock. We can't even kill you."

Robinson laughed between her clenched teeth. "But you all have certainly tried," she muttered.

Little by little, her mouth began to open. Every day, they came to measure to see if it would open wide enough to allow them to operate. "When you can bite a Big Mac," they said, "we're going to the OR." But they warned her that even after surgery she might never swallow again. She hadn't swallowed in more than a year and those muscles had lain dormant all that time. They might never work again.

While waiting for surgery, she almost choked to death twice. The first time, a nurse fed her too fast through the tube in her nose, and then fled the room when she started to choke. Fortunately, a friend visiting from Mississippi saved the day by grabbing a small tube, sticking it between her teeth and suctioning out her throat. The second time, they had to do another emergency tracheotomy. Again, without anesthetic.

After the surgery to fix her breathing, she had surgery to correct the bad bone fusion. They had to go in and take out the metal rod and repair the old fusion. That was a twelve-hour operation. Afterward, the surgeon told her it had been "the most taxing surgery I have ever done. But," he said, "I got you fixed."

"Fixed," of course, was a relative term. She would never be able to turn her head again. Her neck was totally stiff. "You'll have to pivot from your fanny to turn," the surgeon explained.

And for the next ten months, she had to wear a "halo" — a metal contraption that held her head perfectly still in relation to her spine. The halo came off on her fifty-fifth birthday, only to be replaced by a soft collar — pediatric size. (At a slight five feet two inches, Robinson's neck wasn't big enough for an adult collar.)

Finally, after four and a half months in New York, Robinson came home. She hadn't really been back to Coffeeville to stay in almost a year. She brought with her a rigorous therapy regimen. Because her muscles were still spastic, she had to exercise every muscle, every day — even hand exercises for the muscles of her index fingers. But even with all the exercises, she still couldn't raise her arms, her walk was weak, her balance unsteady, and bad weather gave her terrible, arthritis-like pain. She could cook and drive, but she couldn't button buttons, put in her own earrings, or brush the back of her hair. Her hands worked, but not together, so she had to be especially careful when she used a knife. Her biggest fear was falling and "wrecking all of Dr. Stein's hard work."

Still, she was upbeat. "Every day, I sat there. And if I allowed myself to stop and think about it, my body was in agony, my hands were stinging — they stung twenty-four hours a day — my face was hot, and the weather really bothered me. But, do you know, I never noticed it."

She wasn't home long, though, before she had to face yet another problem — a problem of a different sort: Her husband was having an affair. "I had been gone for years and he found him a friend," says Robinson. "He didn't want that woman. He was just lonely." The Robinsons had been married almost forty years. Even worse than the affair, though, was the fact that all of Coffeeville knew about it. "He didn't even bother to hide it in the community," she says. "That really hurt me."

But still she persisted.

A few months later, her house burned down.

She was cooking dinner when she smelled smoke, looked in the garage, and saw her husband's truck on fire. While he tried to battle the blaze with a kitchen fire extinquisher, Robinson limped to the phone and called 911. But the man who answered couldn't understand her because of her high, nasal voice — a legacy of the first, botched bone fusion's effect on her soft palate.

By the time the fire trucks finally arrived, the house — a brand-new one — was a loss. Still, Robinson was philosophical. "Do you know, we walked out of that house and did not pick up one thing," she says, "not one thing. We just walked out."

The Robinsons eventually rebuilt their house, and their marriage. They have thirteen grandchildren; the oldest one is ten. Every Christmas, they throw a party for a hundred friends. And when people in Coffeeville say, "Oh, poor Betty," Robinson replies, "Listen, I can stand. I can take anything that comes. I have already been to hell and back." And when anybody asks her how she's doing, she always looks them in the eye and says, "I'm still here."

It's impossible not to admire someone like Betty Robinson. Even doctors talk about patients like Robinson — and most have had them — with a combination of admiration and amazement. On Robinson's most recent return to New York for a checkup, Dr. Stein spoke for his profession when he told her, "You know, Betty, we're not this good." Our culture celebrates that kind of tenacious perseverence, that persistence in the face of overwhelming adversity, whether the field of struggle is illness or disability, poverty or politics. "I'm still here," is a rallying cry that strikes deep in our survival-instinctive hearts. We root for the Betty Robinsons of the world — and the Sean Laverys, the Jackie Townsends, the Tamara Enochs — because they remind us of what John Gunther called in *Death, Be Not Proud* "the invincibility of the human spirit."

For patients like me who have faced similar (if less extreme) adversity, however, stories like Betty Robinson's, stories of super-human determination and sheer grit, present a daunting challenge: They make it harder for us to ask the question, "When can I stop fighting? Is there a point beyond which I really *shouldn't* be fighting, when it's really not in my best interest to continue the battle? Or should I — should every patient — basically "go for broke"? Follow Betty Robinson's lead and keep on fighting no matter what? If not, then how do I know when to stop? When can I be satisfied that I've really gone as far as I can go, done everything I can do?

Those, unfortunately, were exactly the kinds of questions I was asking after I heard the final word from my operation with Dr. Dolenc. He had not been able to get all the tumor. Indeed, after carefully clearing the cavernous sinus area, he had actually seen additional tumor near the base of my skull but was not able to reach it — something to do with the way he had accessed the area. The surgery had eliminated the most dangerous part of the tumor, all right, but clearly it wasn't the final solution I had hoped for. My blood and bones continued to be a mess, as the remaining tumor continued to pump its chemical static into my system; so I continued to take the supplements that kept me from disintegrating, just as I had been doing for almost twenty years; and wondered, "Now, what?"

Persistence is not easy. Perhaps that's one of the reasons we admire it so much in patients like Betty Robinson. For me, at least, once the threat of imminent death had passed, after the surgery, the only thing that kept me thinking about other options, other procedures, other protocols, was my double vision. I wasn't looking to cure it — I knew it would either clear up on its own or not — but at least it reminded me that I *still had a tumor.* Then, about two months after the operation, the double vision disappeared — and, with it, any determination I had to pursue other possible solutions. For the first time in years, I didn't *have* to think about my tumor, so I didn't. I put the whole thing out of my head, so to speak, even though I knew it was still there, still growing. Denial wasn't just easy, it wasn't just tempting, it was virtually irresistible.

The same is true for most patients. When a disease reaches a crisis point, when life itself is in the balance, it's easy to commit all one's emotional resources to the fight against it. Indeed, it's hard to think about anything else. After the crisis has passed, however, most people don't want to think about their problems, and for the first time in years, perhaps, they don't have to, because they don't have the pain or the limp or the weakness or the slur or the double vision to remind them.

In other words, persistence is hardest when it's needed most. To rally for the big operation, or persist in the search for the right doctor for a one-time procedure, is relatively easy. To persist in the face of a chronic, episodic illness like mine, one that stretches over decades and involves numerous operations and countless complications, isn't. That's when the need to monitor both the disease and medical developments relating to it requires either extraordinary discipline or out-and-out obsession.

Unfortunately, I had neither. And for almost a year, I barely thought about my tumor. I wrote another book with Steve, worked on the house in South Carolina, and lived as though I would never be sick again, in a torpor of denial that even periodic trips to Charlottesville for checkups couldn't penetrate.

But, of course, like Betty Robinson, I *was* sick again.

Like Robinson's, my ordeal (or at least the next round of it) began with a trip to the dentist. I had noticed a strange lump on my lower gum and asked the dentist to identify it. When she couldn't, she referred me to an oral surgeon to have it removed. It's a sign of how oblivious I had grown that during the week we waited for the pathology report, I was not especially anxious.

I should have been. It was, indeed, a tumor, an enchondroma, to be specific, also known simply as a "brown tumor." Of course, it wasn't long before I noticed a pain in my bones when I shook hands with people. As my mind flashed back to law school, metafractures, and useless crutches, I had this horrendous sinking feeling: Was the whole, baroque-ugly tale beginning all over again?

When I rushed back to Charlottesville, they told me I would need *another operation.*

Not brain surgery, this time. Throat surgery. Two decades of chemical chaos in my blood had finally taken their toll on my parathyroid glands. Instead of the pea-sized glands dispensing the tiny amounts of hormone into the bloodstream they were supposed to be, mine had grown into bloated, golf-ball-sized hormone gushers. The resulting overflow of parathyroid hormone was wreaking all kinds of havoc on my bones, of which the brown tumors were only the most visible symptom. If I didn't have the operation, both the pain and the tumors would get worse.

I had the operation. The surgeon slit my throat — literally — took out the offending glands, then placed some smaller, appropriately sized pieces of gland in my forearm. The idea, improbable as it sounds, was that the pieces of gland would quickly develop blood supplies and prosper in their new location, freeing me of the need to supply parathyroid hormone artificially (as diabetics supply their own insulin) for the rest of my life.

The operation went well enough, but the recovery turned out to be a catalog of woes worthy of Betty Robinson. After years of too much calcium in my blood (but not enough phosphorus for my bones to absorb the calcium), suddenly there was none. Caught in this chemical whiplash, my body exploded in a cacophony of bizarre symptoms: strange tinglings, odd reflexes, inexplicable muscle spasms. I heard things, saw things, felt things, that didn't exist. The doctors dripped bag after bag of calcium into my veins, but it just seemed to disappear, so hungry were my bones for the stuff after twenty years of doing without.

Eventually, however, the bones drank their fill and the new

glands in my arm kicked in. The brown tumors dissolved and the pain in my hand went away. I came home from the hospital with stitches in my neck and forearm. By the time they were gone, I had forgotten about the tumor in my head yet again.

Until the first seizure.

It was almost two years after the brain surgery with Dr. Dolenc. So long that I didn't recognize the strange sensation at first — the sense of dislocation, removal, déjà vu. I was grocery shopping when it happened, pushing the cart and then jumping on the back for a few seconds of free flight — an old habit from childhood. Then, suddenly, I wasn't there. Or I wasn't *all* there. At the same time, a brief snatch of music I didn't recognize floated through my head. Dr. Hilal used to call these brief episodes of altered reality "seizures," but "spells" always seemed more descriptive to me. By whatever name, it was the first one in two years. The tumor was back.

Now what?

Part of me, of course, wanted to answer "nothing" — declare the battle a victory and go home. I had been fighting this tumor for twenty years — the last eight of them under a three-month death sentence. I had done pretty well, all things considered. Enough was enough. The mere thought of another round of hospital waiting rooms and grave-faced doctors made me tired. Very tired. Bone tired. Just because I didn't want to fight to the last breath like Betty Robinson, did that make me a quitter?

Besides, what more *could* I do? In those twenty years, I had been everywhere, seen everyone. I had a whole separate Rolodex for doctors. My brain had been photographed more often than Princess Di. Hadn't I gone as far as I could go, done everything I could do?

Actually, no. Any patient who claims that he's done *everything* he can do is probably lying, at least to himself. Because "everything" is a constantly changing set. What was "everything" yesterday, is not "everything" today. I, of all people, should have known that. In 1986, my tumor was officially "inoperable." *Everybody* said so. In 1991, it was operable. From lung transplants to radiosurgery to immunotherapy, medical knowledge is always bounding ahead. So, every day taken back from death is another opportunity for new cures, new drugs, new procedures to emerge. As one doctor told me, "What is not known about medicine far exceeds what is known."

There is, for example, emerging evidence that the immune system can "learn," building up its resistance to diseases, even cancer, over time (giving biological gravity to the old saw, "Whatever doesn't kill me, makes me stronger"). What all this means, as Betty Robinson, Tamara Enoch, Phyllis Kerr, and others have discovered, is that a string of stalemates can add up to a victory. "Every year they learn more things," says Kerr, "and every year is a year that I never had before."

All of those patients would agree, however, that it takes more than just grit and determination to string those stalemates together; it takes more than a special kind of patient to make these slow-motion miracles happen. It takes a special kind of doctor.

A doctor like Mary Lee Vance.

Surgeons are great and I've had some great ones. But, by and large, doctors who "heal with steel" are not characterologically suited to treating chronic illness. By nature, they are problem solvers, not managers; go-getters, not cheerleaders. They tend to be impatient, rather than persistent; decisive rather than determined. And they detest stalemates. One of the things that attracts them to surgery in the first place is the do-something, make-a-difference, before-and-after nature of the work. The most common complaint about surgeons from patients is that they simply are not around enough. Many patients don't meet their surgeons until the day before their operation; some not until the morning of. The reason is simple: Most surgeons don't treat patients, they treat problems. One doctor I spoke to characterized their attitude this way: "A car mechanic doesn't need to get to know the owner of the car to fix a knock in the engine."

Thoughtful surgeons (and there are lots of them) will acknowledge, however, that many problems in medicine don't lend themselves to the kind of black-and-white "fix" that surgery celebrates. And there are other kinds of problems for which surgery is only part of the solution, not all. My case is a perfect example. Two brain surgeries, two embolizations, and a parathyroidectomy — a lot of surgery — had not solved my problem. Most of it had helped; some of it, certainly, had averted more serious crises, but the problem in my blood and bones required a different kind of solution from a different kind of doctor.

A doctor like Mary Lee Vance.

I first met Dr. Vance when I came to U.V.A. to do the surgery with Dr. Dolenc. Thanks to the research Steve and I had done for the first edition of *The Best Doctors in America,* I already knew that she was one of the country's leading endocrinologists, doctors who specialize in hormonal secretions — not exactly a flashy niche in the edifice of medicine. The diseases she dealt with tended to be long-term — like hormone imbalances — diseases that erode life slowly from within, rather than extinguish it quickly in a catastrophic coup de grâce. She was used to the long haul, the incremental improvements of long-term therapy, the stringing together of small victories, rather than the heroic, twelve-hour, life-saving extravaganzas of surgery.

She was also used to patients. After my surgery, she was the one who took over "caring" when Dr. Dolenc jetted off to the next international conference, the next brilliant performance in the next operating theater. Although raised in the heady, effervescent atmosphere of New Orleans, she could be spare and formal at times (I never could get her to call me anything but "Mr. Smith"), yet there was something about her attention to human needs, her attunement to suffering, her genuine joy at every success, that suggested more a Mardi Gras float than a Shaker chair. She spent more time with her patients than any doctor I had ever seen — and I had seen my share. She came in the mornings surrounded by students. She came in the afternoons with other doctors. She came in the evenings by herself for one last check of the charts, the latest lab results, the next day's tests. She understood that the hardest part of catastrophic illness isn't the catastrophe, it's what the catastrophe does to your daily life. So she became a part of your daily life. She came on weekends. She came on holidays (I never figured out where she fit a personal life) — moved in equal parts by professional conscientiousness, intellectual rigor, inexhaustible compassion, and, most important, a sheer, innate curiosity, a love of puzzles. To her, all patients were puzzles. Puzzles with lives, and loved ones.

And I was the biggest puzzle she had seen in a while.

Dr. Vance was the one who supervised my periodic checkups, testing to see how the surgery had affected my blood and bones, "inferring" the status of my tumor from the levels of calcium and phosophorus in my blood. She was the one who told me it was time to have my bloated parathyroid glands removed, and, afterward, shepherded me through the strange array of afflictions as my body adjusted to its new, radically altered chemical environment.

It was Dr. Vance who, when I rushed back to Charlottesville after the first seizure, sat me down (calmed me down) and reviewed all the possible new treatments for tumors like mine. She was the one who suggested the possibility that my tumor, like other neuroendocrine tumors, might respond to hormone treatment. She had, in fact, had great success treating pituitary tumors with an experimental artifical hormone called somatostatin, a hormone naturally present in the body in tiny amounts that suppresses growth of all kinds. She had used it to treat patients with acromegalia, a rare growth disorder that causes enlarged extremities, facial deformations, and a litany of internal problems that typically lead to early death (as it did for the most famous acromegalic, professional wrestler Andre the Giant).

It was Dr. Vance who, on nothing more than a hunch, sent me to a doctor at Ohio State to have my tumor "scanned" for somatostatin receptors — the chemical keyholes for which hormones are the key. If the tumor did have receptors, theoretically at least, heavy and continuous doses of somatostatin might suppress its growth — might even reverse it. In some of her acromegalic patients, the tumors had disappeared. But I didn't let myself think about that.

TWENTY-ONE

Drawing the Line

DR. VANCE MADE it easy for me. By giving me something to hook my hope to, she made it possible to keep fighting at a time when, without that hope, it would have been so much easier to give up. Because of her, I never had to face the questions that raced through my mind that day in the grocery store when the seizures reappeared: Have I done everything I can? Have I gone far enough? Can I stop now?

But what about patients who aren't as lucky as I was? What about patients who don't have a Dr. Vance to throw them a lifeline but who are still, like Betty Robinson, "determined to live"? How do they know they've gone far enough? Is it possible to go too far? To "chase after rainbows that aren't really there," as Dr. Sorrell says? When does healthy persistence become unhealthy obsession?

Many patients who don't find the hope they're looking for in mainstream medicine eventually look to alternative or nontraditional therapies. At various times over the last twenty years, when traditional medicine looked like a dead end, I explored self-hypnosis, visualization, and macrobiotics. I'll never forget the visit of a macrobiotic "expert" to our apartment in New York. I told her over the phone that I had been diagnosed with a brain tumor. "We've had very good results with brain tumors," she assured me. "Let me examine you." When I greeted her at the door, she looked deeply into my eyes and said, "Yes, I can *see* the tumor." Then she walked to the kitchen and, after surveying the shelves, identified the source of my problem: "Too much chocolate."

At another point, Steve contacted a leading specialist in traditional Chinese medicine from Beijing who happened to be spending a year at M.G.H. in Boston. What kind of herbal cures did he recommend for brain tumors? Steve asked.

"We don't have any," the man replied.

"Then what do you recommend?"

"Surgery," he said.

"But what did they do in China traditionally, before they had surgery?" Steve pressed.

"They died," he said.

There is nothing funny, however, about the woman in Colorado who recovered from breast cancer using a combination of yoga and T'ai Chi. Or the filmmaker in New York City who, upon being diagnosed with terminal cancer, went to Maine, meditated, and drank concentrated doses of blenderized vegetables. When she returned to her doctor, "there was no evidence of disease." And there's certainly nothing funny about the nine-year-old boy with a huge astrocytoma in his brain that he made go away by "visualizing" his own white blood cells eating it up.

Alternative medicine — or nontraditional medicine or "fringe" medicine — is a very big tent. It covers visualization, meditation, yoga, diet, therapeutic touch, homeopathy, shark cartilage, various vegetable concoctions, vitamin megadoses, etc. It draws patients from every stratum of society. A prominent alternative medicine doctor in New York says of his clientele, "They range from Arkansas farmers to statesmen and all variations in between. Hollywood people, salesmen from Omaha, insurance executives, health-food-store owners. The one common denominator is they tend to be very independent." A more traditional doctor characterizes their "common denominator" in a slightly different way. "They're all just trying to hold on," she says.

Under the "big top" of alternative medicine, all kinds of salesmen hawk their wares, from the serious to the crackpot. From the psychologist at the Menninger Clinic who only treats children using visual imagery, to the diet gurus who ply the late-night channel surf with infomercials and extravagant promises. And it isn't always easy to tell them apart. One of the most respected practitioners in the field of alternative medicine, Dr. Nicholas Gonzalez, offers his patients a program of nutritional cancer therapies based on the supposed anticancer effects of pancreatic enzymes. His program is based, in turn, on the work of a doctor "who spent twenty-five years treating patients," says Gonzalez. "On our first review of his records, which took five years, we studied the effectiveness of his program in twenty-six different types of cancer, from acute leukemias to pancreatic cancer, all of which we documented. So we know that it works on a variety of different cancers."

Who is this pathbreaking doctor, and where did he do his research? Mayo? Sloan-Kettering? M. D. Anderson? NIH?

Actually, he's an eccentric dentist who worked out of a storefront office in rural Texas. "He's still alive and still crazy," says Gonzalez. "He's a loon. And he's kind of a recluse; doesn't talk to anyone. I understand he's living with his ninety-year-old mother. Great ideas come out of weird sources."

Perhaps. Apparently the National Institutes of Health think so. Recently, NIH created a department for the study of alternative medicine, "in recognition that there are other influences over health that haven't been part of mainstream medicine." Among the alternative therapies under study: therapeutic touch, prayer, and the Texas dentist's pancreatic enzymes.

Not surprisingly, doctors disagree widely on the effectiveness of these and other alternatives to mainstream medicine. Only rarely are they subjected to the kind of rigorous, double-blind testing that experimental treatments in the mainstream must undergo. And when they are, they tend to fail. Just to pick one example, a study done to test Linus Pauling's famous claims for megadoses of vitamin C in treating cancer concluded that such doses "did not make much difference in the course of the illness."

But what about the stories? What about the woman who cured herself of breast cancer with yoga, the filmmaker who fought her terminal cancer with a trip to Maine, or the boy who visualized his brain tumor away? Dr. Patricia Norris of the Life Sciences Institute of Mind-Body Health in Topeka, Kansas, who treated the last of these, argues that such anecdotal evidence is proof that these therapies work; we just don't yet understand *how* they work. "The bottom line," says Norris, "is that we know that immune cells have receptors for neural transmitters. Anything that the brain can say chemically can be heard by the immune system. In fact, there's such a close link that some of the scientists in this area are saying that the immune system is the part of the brain that travels around. We are just beginning to understand what some of these things are."

Perhaps. But a cancer specialist I spoke to warned against the dangers of taking anecdotal evidence as proof. "We need to remember that only the living speak," says Dr. Robert Oldham, a well-known immunotherapist, formerly of NIH and currently director of the Biological Therapy Institute in Franklin, Tennessee. In other words, for every woman who cures herself with yoga or meditation or trips to Maine, for every child who visualizes away a tumor, there may be hundreds, even thousands of similar patients who tried the same "therapies" *without* success, and are therefore not around to testify to their ineffectiveness.

Doctors may disagree about the effectiveness of alternative medicine, but on one point they are unanimous. "Anything you want to add that makes you feel better is great," says Dr. Gordon

Schwartz, the surgical oncologist, "whether it's prayer or silenium and zinc, anything as long as it's *in addition* to science, not instead of science, I'm all for it. The way I put it to my patients is, 'I'll take all the help I can get.'" Dr. Samuel Klagsbrun, the psychiatrist, *insists* that his patients be "in mainstream therapy and on medication." "If they want to take coffee grounds, laetrile, or any damned thing they want to in addition, I don't say no, but they must be in the hands of a respected oncologist."

Indeed, most patients do both. That woman in Colorado who treated herself with yoga? She did traditional therapy as well. And when the cancer reappeared in her liver five years later, she underwent very aggressive chemotherapy and radiation. The nine-year-old boy with the astrocytoma tried radiation before turning to visualization. Did the radiation make his tumor go away or the visualization, or both? Even the doctor who treated him answers that question cautiously. "I can never say he wouldn't have made it if he hadn't done this," says Patricia Norris, "but I think it greatly increased his chances." That's exactly how Richard Bloch, the tax-consultation mogul and former cancer patient, thinks about his use of visualization. "I can't claim it is what cured me," says Bloch, "but I think it made the difference between success and failure. I was cured with radiation and chemo, but I think visualization is what made the radiation and chemo successful." Bloch doesn't like the terms nontraditional or alternative for therapies like visualization. He prefers to call them "supplemental therapies."

There are dangers, however. In her brain tumor support group, Virginia Andriola has noticed an increased interest in alternative medicine among both patients and their families, and she worries that in some cases it represents "a mistrust of the health care system: patients asking what do the doctors really know?" In addition, because they are often unsupervised, some alternative therapies can make a patient sicker. "When a patient raises the possibility of fringe medicine," says Dr. Murray Brennan, the chairman of surgery at Sloan-Kettering, "I focus on making sure it won't do any harm." For example, if patients want to take massive doses of vitamins — "which I don't believe can be made to show a difference," says Brennan, "because we all know that most of it will be passed out in the urine" — he tells them, "Just don't take so much that you get sick. And if through taking vitamins your head feels better, and that feeling of well-being impacts on how you cope with your tumor, then that was a very good strategy for you."

The greatest concern doctors have, though, is that if conventional medicine doesn't work, patients will buy into the kind of expensive "alternative therapies" that flourish in places like Mexico and the Bahamas — just beyond the reach of the FDA — and are set up specifically for the purpose of separating desperate patients from their money. Dr. William Wood, the surgical oncologist, says patients often ask him about such programs. "They will say they have a cousin who sent them this clipping, and, for a hundred thousand dollars, they can go get worked up and perhaps develop an immunization that will make the tumor go away. And they're all prepared to mortgage the house and go if someone thinks it's going to be to their advantage." "I hate to see people spending their money or running off to Mexico," says Cancer Care's Diane Blum. "I remember years ago I had a patient with lymphoma who had a disease that was really potentially treatable and chose to go to the Bahamas and do one of these alternative things, and the patient died. I mean, that gets scary."

In assessing such programs, Dr. Oldham reminds patients, again, that "only the living speak." "If you go to the laetrile clinics, you will find people down there who believe for all the world that the only reason they are alive is because they got out of the medical system, got down to Mexico, and started taking coffee enemas or laetrile or sheep dust or something. But you don't know how many others went through the same program and were *not* successful and are *not* around to tell you about their bad experiences."

Just as there are wrong *ways* to keep fighting, there are, according to most doctors, wrong reasons. "Sometimes," says Dr. James Cimino, a kidney specialist at Calvary Hospital in the Bronx, "it's the doctor who doesn't want to give up. The patient's survival becomes an ego issue rather than an altruistic issue." According to Cimino, some doctors develop reputations for not giving up easily. "But a doctor who is functioning primarily on an egotistical value system," Cimino cautions, "could subject that patient to undue suffering without realizing it." One doctor told me about a case where a surgeon performed an operation to repair a small abdominal aneurysm in an eighty-year-old man suffering from Alzheimer's disease. "What else besides ego," he asks, "could explain putting an old man with no symptoms in the hospital for weeks, months maybe, to operate on something that wasn't killing him and probably wouldn't for five years?"

But a doctor's ego isn't the only thing that can cause a patient "undue suffering." It can be something as benign as a family's love. Sometimes, it's the patient's family and friends who want to keep fighting, not the patient. They want "the best care for their loved one." They want him or her to "have every chance." Only the loved one doesn't *want* any more care or any more chances. "It's a very, very difficult line to draw," says Virginia Andriola of the brain tumor support group at Columbia-Presbyterian, "between what patients want for themselves and what their loved ones want for them. It comes up all the time in different ways. Where do you push and where do you stop and where do you let the patient make the decision for herself? Questions like that can cause a lot of friction and stress between family members."

Andriola remembers a young man who kept "dragging his mother from place to place." She had a brain tumor and "he wanted her to deal with it aggressively, but she didn't want to. He kept saying he wanted her to have every chance." The conflict broke into the open when he found an experimental treatment in Houston that he wanted her to try. "He had done all this research," Andriola recalls, "and thought that this was going to make all the difference." But his mother didn't want to do it. She wanted to stick with the conventional treatment she was receiving at Columbia-Presbyterian. Her doctors assured her they were doing everything that could be done and she was "getting along pretty well on her own," says Andriola. "Her son wanted her to go that one extra step, but she didn't want to."

The right time to stop fighting may not be clear, but one thing is clear: The person who should make that decision is the patient. While it's perfectly appropriate for loved ones to "give a patient encouragement in their fight," says Andriola, "they need to remember that it's still the patient's life, still their body, still their illness."

When is it "right" to keep fighting? The experts seem to agree that persistence based on a realistic assessment — even an optimistic assessment — of a patient's condition (prognosis, options for treatment, chances of success) is good. But persistence based on denial is not. How can a patient (or a patient's family) tell the difference? Dr. William Wood has an unusual strategy for making that distinction: He tells his breast surgery patients to "make preparations for dying." "First, I tell them they need to be legally ready to die," says Wood, "make out their will, that sort of thing. Second, they need to have their family relationships in order. If there is some member of the family from whom they feel estranged, they need to go to that person and rebuild those bridges. And, third, they need to be spiritually ready to die. If they are not in a relationship with their God and they realize that they want to be, this is the time to do it."

Why all these preparations for death? Because "preparation is the other side of persistence" says Wood. "When people have a recurrent disease, they very often get into a mind game with themselves. They decide that they can't make out their will or reconcile with family members because, if they do, that would be giving up. That would be admitting that they are going to die. So to be brave, to be macho, to be optimistic, they don't do those things." Wanting to fight death with every available means is one thing; wanting to run from death and hide behind yet another treatment — any treatment — is something else. "Decisions about care should be made out of a determination to live," says Wood, "not out of a fear of dying, or a denial of death."

Ultimately, the question a patient has to ask is not "*Can* I keep fighting?" but instead "*Why* do I want to keep fighting?" "What am I fighting *for*?" This is where that simple, stirring affirmation "I'm still here" gets complicated. In our minds and in our popular culture, the emphasis is almost always on "still." We admire someone who is *still* here after going through what Betty Robinson went through. The longer and more agonizing the ordeal, the braver and more triumphant it sounds: "I'm *still* here." What the experts are saying is that patients need to put an equal emphasis on "here" — "I'm still *here*" — and ask themselves, "Where is 'here'?"

No one has more of a right to crow "I'm still here" than Daniel Carrey, a ninety-year-old man who was admitted to the hospital with end-stage kidney disease. He had no kidney function at all. He had a previous history of coronary artery problems, including open heart surgery when he was a mere eighty. His blood pressure was low. He was septic. He had multiple organ system failures. And on top of all that, he had pneumonia, which was what had brought him to the ER. Even before this emergency, Carrey was alive only because of a catheter in his abdomen through which constant dialysis was done at home. Dazed and confused in intensive care, he was made "DNR" — "Do Not Resuscitate" — several times; that is, doctors decided that if he stopped breathing or his heart stopped beating, they would make no effort to revive him.

"Everybody had thrown in the towel on him," Carrey's doctor told me, "but I didn't, and he didn't. With some encouragement from me, he persisted."

A triumph? Not everyone thought so. Most of Carrey's family

members and friends, even the nurses in the intensive care unit, "didn't feel it was worth it," his doctor recalls. "They were all feeling the same thing: He's lethargic, his blood pressure is falling, he's septic, he's dying, he's ninety, *leave him alone.*" By the doctor's own admission, "ninety-nine percent" of his colleagues in the hospital felt the same way. "I had a lot of pressure put on me," he recalls. The pressure only intensified when he put a feeding tube in the man's neck. "I had doctors and nurses coming up to me saying, 'What are you doing? Why are you doing it? He's dying. Leave him alone.' But we hung in there."

After six weeks of intensive care, Carrey did eventually leave the hospital alive. He went home to round-the-clock nursing care, physical therapy, and perpetual dialysis. He can't walk. After months of intravenous feedings, he has graduated to oatmeal and pureed chicken soup.

But he's "still here."

Is that something to celebrate? His daughter (the one family member who wasn't ready to throw in the towel) certainly thinks so. "I really feel that he's going to make it to his ninety-first birthday," she says. "He just *has* to." Carrey's doctor describes the case as "one of the nicer turnarounds in my twenty-six years of practice." The patient himself isn't saying much.

Is the fact that Daniel Carrey is talking at all — the fact that he's "still here" — a triumph? Joan Teckman, the young swimmer who was diagnosed with cystic fibrosis, wouldn't think so. Before her double lung transplant, people laughed at her because she planned to stay in her own condo after the operation. "Everybody else who was recovering from a transplant lived in their family's house and their moms put their food in front of them," she recalls, "but I wouldn't let my mom do that for me. I had to keep my independence, and if I couldn't keep my independence, I didn't want to be alive."

Another patient who wouldn't find Carrey's story a triumph is the woman with lung cancer who told me, "As long as I can still enjoy a good meal, I'm not ready to check out." She could have coped with Carrey's immobility — she herself had metastases in her spine and no function in her legs — but not his diet of oatmeal and pureed chicken soup. "Everybody draws the line in a different place," says Dr. David Peretz, the psychiatrist, "the line between what is worth fighting for and what is not. The line beyond which they're no longer willing to carry on the battle."

"Some people are tenacious and won't take no for an answer," says Dr. Jeffrey Glassroth, the pulmonary specialist at Northwestern. "They will be fighting and taking an experimental drug up to their last breath. They will do absolutely everything they can, even to the point where the treatment is worse than the disease, if that's possible. While others really have come to terms, made peace with their illnesses, and for whatever reason don't want to undergo extreme treatments." According to Virginia Andriola, men and women tend to draw their lines in different places. "Men have a tendency to say, 'We're going to beat this no matter what,'" says Andriola, "while women have a tendency to say, 'I want the best quality of life.'"

More and more, doctors are responding to the lines their patients draw. "We've lived for years with this idea that if you cure the disease, don't bother me with this other stuff," says Diane Blum of Cancer Care. "Now we're becoming much more sophisticated. We are beginning to understand that, yes, cure is good — that's what we're aiming for — but we also have to think about quality of life." Doctors talk about these lines in terms of "futility" — when is it futile to continue treatments? — but more and more they define futility in terms of quality of life rather than merely in terms of statistical probability; in terms of what quality of life is acceptable *to this patient*. "Once the patient makes that decision," says Dr. Andrew von Eschenbach, "then I think you have to support them in that. They have the right to say enough's enough, I'm not going to continue on."

Where *should* a patient draw the line? Unfortunately, there is no easy rule. "You have to do everything according to your own way of doing it," says Alice Trillin. Whether the question is "Do I pursue alternative therapies?" or "Who decides when enough is enough?" or "When should I stop fighting?" the most important consideration, as Trillin says, is *not to turn yourself into someone else*. Because then, in a way, the disease would be defeating you."

That's where Trillin drew the line. "I was always so conscious of that," she says. " 'Please don't let this whole ordeal turn me into someone else, a frightened person, an irrational person, a person who's really out of control.' For me, that was the most terrifying prospect."

That's where I drew the line, too.

Would I pursue a treatment that would leave me sightless or speechless, or steal my memory? Would I fight for life at any price? I had friends who wondered why I would risk an experimental hormone treatment when my only complaint was an occasional seizure. After all, the seizures weren't frequent, they didn't last long, they weren't painful. My scans didn't show any imminent threat from the tumor. Did I really want to venture into uncharted water with so little at stake? My response was always the same: "Imagine that someone out there wants to kill you. In fact, they've already tried and failed — twice. You think you're in the clear for a while, and then you go to your mailbox one day and there's a postcard from the would-be killer. "I'm still here," it says. "And today could be the day." And then postcards like that start arriving every couple of days, sometimes two a day.

That's what those seizures were: postcards from the edge. No, they didn't last long; they weren't painful; they didn't interfere with my routine. But by reminding me daily of how close to the edge I was, they were changing me slowly but inexorably into someone else: a man on the run.

That's why I was willing to risk the unknown consequences of hormone therapy. That's why I had been willing to risk so much — speech, sight, memory — in the surgery with Dr. Dolenc.

And would again. I was hoping for the same thing from all of them: Dr. Hilal, Dr. Dolenc, Dr. Vance. Deliverance. Deliverance from the tumor, of course, if possible; temporary deliverance from its effects, if not; but most of all, deliverance from *fear*— the daily fear that today, or the next day, with the next seizure or the next rush to the hospital, I would yet again have to face all the same questions about life and death and dying, and where to draw the line. I was tired of living every day on the edge of my mortality. More than anything — more than life itself, I guess — I wanted a life without fear.

So finally, in addition to an emphasis on "still" and "here," there also needs to be an emphasis on "I" — "*I'm* still here." No matter how brave and furious the battle, no matter how tolerable the quality of life when the struggle is over, if the disease *or* the treatment changes me in the process, makes me act like someone other than who I am, if it "coerces me out of my identity," to borrow Seamus Heaney's phrase, then *someone* may be "still here," but that someone is not "I." And, as Alice Trillin says, "If you become a different person, you've really lost the battle anyway."

TWENTY-TWO

Hope

JOHN GROUT WAS diagnosed in 1994 with an incurable and always fatal disease. When he looked for treatments, he found only a few drugs, and those would only delay the symptoms, not alter the end. And an ugly end it was: immune system malfunction, respiratory and coronary breakdown, multiple system failures — "a pretty nasty way to go," as one of his doctors described it. The normal progression of the disease was about ten years, although it varied widely from patient to patient. Grout, a chemist by training, buried himself in medical books and journals, searching desperately for the clue that everyone else had missed. But no matter where he turned, the answers were always the same: No cure. *Always* fatal.

Was his a "hopeless" case? Is there such a thing as a hopeless case? "I don't ever say that anything is totally one hundred percent hopeless," says Dr. Andrew von Eschenbach, the urologic oncologist; and most of the doctors I spoke to agreed. They're careful not to give patients false hope and they think difficult "quality of life" questions need to be asked before pursuing endgame therapies, but most don't believe any case is truly, utterly, ir-retrievably hopeless. They know better. They've been proved wrong too often. "I've seen a lot of people who go on a lot longer than you thought they would and you can't really explain it," says Dr. Edward Rosenow, the head of thoracic diseases at the Mayo Clinic. "We look for every possible explanation," says Dr. Dorothy White, the pulmonary specialist at Sloan-Kettering, "but some-times we don't find any and we're just left with being very de-lighted that someone has done it." "We've had people who've had some pretty spectacular regression," says Dr. W. Marston Linehan, the head of urologic oncology at NIH, "long-term and complete remissions. So we're very careful about using the word hopeless." "There *are* miracles," concedes Dr. Thomas Petty, the pulmo-nologist at Denver's Presbyterian–St. Luke's Hospital. "There are these rare — hard to document but a few have been documented — cases of spontaneous remission from cancer. There's got to be some immune mechanism that explains them."

Perhaps. But until that mechanism is explained, they remain "miracles."

No one knows more about hope and hopelessness than Dr. James Cimino. He is the director of a hospital specifically set up for "hopeless cases," Calvary Hospital in the Bronx, an institu-tion better known by its street name, "The Hospital of the Dy-ing." The name dates from a previous era in medicine, but is still richly deserved. Calvary treats only advanced cancer patients who require acute care. Of all the elderly and terminally ill patients who check into Calvary, only 7 percent ever check out. "Of every one hundred lung cancer patients that are here at any one time," says Cimino, "all but two will be gone within a year."

How does Cimino offer hope to his patients, many of whom know Calvary's reputation before they arrive, and all of whom, Cimino admits, "certainly know that very few people who come here are rehabilitated to the point of having a normal quality of life again"? What does he tell the lung cancer patient who says, "Doctor, my daughter's getting married in six months and I really would like to stay alive that long. Do you think I'll still be here?"

"I tell them, 'If you had come to me six months ago, I wouldn't have been able to tell you with any assurance that you would still be alive today,'" says Cimino. "'But here you are. It is true that most patients with your kind of cancer don't survive for two years, but some people have fooled us." In other words, while it's true that only 2 percent of Calvary's lung cancer patients will survive a year, no one knows *which* 2 percent. For patients at the Hospital of the Dying, that 2 percent is the margin of hope. "I try never to dash hope," says Cimino. "I try to always leave an opening."

An "opening" like the fact that different people react differently to the same diseases — and to the same treatments. "You can hope you're one of the lucky ones," says Cimino. "It's *always* reasonable to hope." Whether the lucky ones are lucky because their immune systems are different or because the virus (or cancer or whatever) they're fighting is different, is a question medical science hasn't answered yet. "All we know," admits Dr. Henry Masur, the chief of critical care medicine at NIH and a prominent AIDS specialist, "is that there are some patients who just do better, last longer, with the same treatment. And that's true of even the most serious, seemingly hopeless afflictions."

Like malignant melanoma. Widely feared as one of the most aggressive, intractable, incurable, and fatal of cancers, this skin cancer is also "one of those unusual tumors to which we know the body can have an immune response," says Dr. Murray Brennan, the head of surgery at Sloan-Kettering. "So there are some patients who have an immune response that actually makes their tumor go away. It's very uncommon, but it does happen." Brennan cites the case of a man who came to him in 1980 with malignant melanoma that involved both his skin and his lymph nodes. Brennan operated on the man despite the fact that "in most people, his condition would have been considered incurable." Seven years later, the man had a craniotomy to remove a tumor from his head; the melanoma had spread to his brain. The very next year, Brennan operated on him again for a bleeding tumor in his stomach; the melanoma had metastasized to his gut. The man is sixty now, still alive — and with no sign of tumor.

"We assumed there were residual tumor cells elsewhere in his body, but his system must have coped with them," says Brennan, shaking his head ever so slightly. (Brennan makes the point, however, that the man did not just "will" his cancer away. Indeed, his aggressive pursuit of treatment for the tumors that were putting his life at risk might have "made it possible for his body to take care of the rest." Dr. Cimino tells his patients, "If you can do something to save yourself, do it.")

Another "opening" for hope is the furious pace of medical innovation. "Just in my professional lifetime," says Cimino, "we have seen dramatic changes in terms of life expectancy in three areas: kidney failure, coronary artery disease, and organ transplant. When I graduated in 1954, patients with those problems didn't have a future. Now they do. It's almost like having lived through the antibiotic era."

Dr. Joel Cooper, who made his reputation transplanting one, then two lungs, has more recently taken the transplant revolution in the opposite direction — saving organs — with his new lung reduction procedure. When asked about "hopeless cases," Cooper cites cystic fibrosis patients. "These are people who have a genetic deficiency, and when I was in medical school, we assumed they'd all die by the age of eight. Now, with transplants, half of them live to age twenty-five."

In the meantime, advances in dealing with transplant disease have made an "opening for hope" that used to be available only to the most robust candidates, or only to those with certain kinds of afflictions, available to a broader range of patients. "It used to be said that we wouldn't transplant anybody over the age of forty or forty-five," says Dr. Michael Sorrell, the liver transplant specialist at the University of Nebraska. "Now, we transplant people in their sixties routinely, and they do very well."

But that, says Cooper, is only the beginning of what is possible in the field of transplantation. "We are working to solve the xeno-graft problem," says Cooper, "namely using organs from pigs or chimpanzees in humans. That could happen in my lifetime."

Not all the revolutionary changes in medicine are ushered in on banner headlines, however. Sometimes, they are the result of small, almost imperceptible advances in technology. The best example comes from Dr. Cimino's own field, chronic renal failure. Without the invention of Teflon (best known as a nonstick cooking sur-face), doctors like Cimino wouldn't have the special tubes that allow them to put patients on dialysis for long periods without re-sorting to powerful anticoagulating drugs. And what did patients with chronic renal failure do before Teflon made hemodialysis widely available? "They just died," says Cimino.

But what about medical advances dealing with tumors like mine? What is on the horizon in the treatment of soft tissue tu-mors (like hemangiopericytomas) in "unremovable places" (like the cavernous sinus)? In addition to hormone therapies like the one I'm on, there is an array of "possibilities" out there: the identification of proteins that inhibit a tumor's ability to develop a blood supply; new, more refined forms of embolization so that chemotherapeutic "bombs" can be delivered directly to a tumor's doorstep; new methods of "marking" tumor cells to make them more visible and more vulnerable, either to the body's own de-fenses or to outside agents like radiation. Surgical techniques are also improving. Radiosurgery continues to undergo refinements. Doctors at one hospital in Boston are now doing MRI-guided surgery. Who knows how many of these methods will prove suc-cessful. But it only takes one. And that one is *my* margin of hope.

Certainly, stranger, more miraculous things have happened —

are happening — every day in medicine. An aneurysm patient at my old hospital, Columbia-Presbyterian, was recently operated on using a new method called "circulatory arrest." "What we actually did," one of her doctors told me, "was cool the patient and then stop her circulation while we worked on her brain arteries." But didn't that mean the patient was dead? "Yes," said the doctor without skipping a beat, "the patient was dead, essentially dead. But then we brought her back to life. Today, she's sitting up talking."

Ten years ago, even five, that kind of medical technology would have been indistinguishable from a miracle.

Nowhere have the changes been more revolutionary, more breathtakingly dramatic, more "miraculous," than in the treatment of cancer.

Cancer was once thought hopeless. Indeed, there was a time when cancer defined hopeless. So potent a death sentence was it that some people wouldn't even utter the word. Today, while still a formidable and terrifying disease, cancer is no longer the one-way ticket it used to be. "Twenty-five years ago most childhood cancers were fatal," says Dr. Philip Pizzo, the head of pediatric medicine at NCI, "but today, if you look at the average, sixty percent of childhood cancers are now just about curable." Indeed, if cervical cancer and common skin cancers are excluded, almost 55 percent of *all* cancers are curable. Purely by the numbers, cancer is more curable than emphysema and certainly more curable than arthritis, for which there is still no known cure.

Like many doctors, Dr. W. Marston Linehan, the eminent kidney cancer specialist, has been tempted by hopelessness. "You see this cancer and what it does to people," says Linehan, "and there are times when you feel like those physicians must have felt with the plague." Yet when he looks at the "biomedical revolution that we're all part of," he can't help but be optimistic. Recently, scientists at Johns Hopkins developed a way to detect bladder cancer in the urine by gene analysis. A similar test for kidney cancer won't be far behind. Once the disease is detectable early, says Linehan, "we can cure people. Today if someone goes to the doctor and their disease is advanced, only ten percent will survive two years. With early detection, we can cure up to ninety-five percent. So, yes, I'm personally very hopeful and optimistic."

So is Dr. William Wood, the surgical oncologist. Like Dr. Linehan, he finds it impossible to look at the developments in gene therapy and immunotherapy and not be hopeful. "We're already putting marker genes in sickle cell patients," says Wood, "and we're on the verge of genetic manipulation of some of these breast tumors." In fact, says Wood, he hopes to offer a genetic treatment for breast cancer "in the very near future." Immunotherapies — therapies that direct the body's own immune system to attack a cancer — "have had their greatest successes in kidney cancer and melanomas," according to Dr. Robert Oldham, a well-known immunotherapist, "and some forms of leukemia and lymphoma are responding well."

Where once there was no hope, now, it seems, there is hope everywhere one looks. Researchers have recently discovered that there is biologic variability to cancers under the microscope; a biologic variability that plays a major role in the course of the disease. There's also evidence that not all cancers, even though they come from the same organ, are, in fact, the same. In other words, new truths lie out there undiscovered. That which we think we know best, we will find we don't know at all. The settled will be unsettled, the hopeless made hopeful, the incurable cured.

Slowly, very slowly, the new reality is changing the way the public — and patients — think about cancer. As early as 1974, Calvary's Dr. Cimino argued that cancer was a chronic disease, not a terminal one. "The reason that people fear cancer so much is that they think of it as terminal immediately," says Cimino, "and now the fact that you can live with it for a long while and sometimes longer than, for example, patients who have acute coronaries could live, that has given people hope that they didn't have before." Back in 1974, Cimino was the lone hopeful voice in a wilderness of despair. Now, he notices many of his cancer patients believe "in the back of their minds, even though they don't articulate it, that there's a chance they're going to, if not be cured, at least live with the disease. Many of them believe they can live."

And what of the unspeakable tragedy of AIDS?

If ever there was a truly hopeless case, this would seem to be it. "AIDS is seen as a universal death sentence," says Dr. Samuel Klagsbrun, the psychiatrist at Four Winds Hospital. "It's not a matter of beating it. With AIDS, no one believes you can beat it, so there is no notion of hope."

"But," says Klagsbrun, "cancer *used* to be that way."

AIDS is the new cancer. The latest in a long line of fearful diseases that once spelled automatic, inexorable, and usually agonizing death. Dr. Cimino remembers a time when his patients in a Buffalo public hospital serving mostly low-income neighborhoods "were more frightened if I told them that their loved one had tuberculosis. If I said, 'I'm sorry to say that the lesion on the lung is cancer,' they would say, 'Oh, thank God, I was afraid it was TB.'" Before tuberculosis, it was cholera, or typhoid, or bubonic plague.

Today, it's AIDS. Dr. Dorothy White, the pulmonologist, says that at her hospital, Memorial Sloan-Kettering, where patients with all kinds of afflictions wait together in large waiting rooms, "the cancer patients don't like to sit near the AIDS patients because the AIDS patients depress them." Several doctors told me that most of their patients today, if given a choice, would prefer to have cancer rather than AIDS, "even though there is a whole spectrum of cancers that are much worse than AIDS." "The existence of AIDS is reshaping our attitude toward cancer," says

Dr. Cimino. "Now that we've got this other huge disease out there that's even worse, that doesn't allow for hope, patients who get cancer think to themselves, 'At least it's not AIDS.'"

The stigma that used to attach to cancer now attaches to AIDS. Twenty years ago obituaries would say, "Died after a long illness," when they should have said simply, "Died of cancer." Now they say, "Died of pneumonia," when they mean, "Died of AIDS." Dr. White remembers a time when nobody talked about "Mom's problem," even though Mom was being treated at Memorial Sloan-Kettering, a center that treated only cancer patients. "If anything," says White, "AIDS patients have it worse." During the first years of the epidemic, many patients arrived at Memorial "with no family support at all. No one knew that they had HIV or AIDS or that they had a risk factor for it, and they were afraid. So they would come in with these desperate pneumonias because they had tried to stay out of the hospital or away from medical care as long as possible because they didn't want people to find out that they had it. And even then, sometimes, they wouldn't tell their families, and we would have to tell the mother or whoever, 'Yes, this patient has a serious pneumonia, and it is a pneumonia seen with AIDS.'"

Although many AIDS patients make up for estrangement from their biological families with strong "adoptive" families and friends (as well as an extraordinary network of support organizations — "a paradigm of human compassion," one doctor called it), few can escape the stigma of their disease. Many of the afflictions that their flesh is heir to, like Kaposi's sarcoma, are public badges, "scarlet lesions." Cancer Care's Diane Blum concedes reluctantly that "AIDS is one of the best things that ever happened to cancer. Cancer has lost some of its stigma because AIDS has so much more of a stigma. The people who get AIDS, for the most part, are people who have been somewhat stigmatized in society anyway."

So the AIDS patient faces not just a medical death sentence, but public scorn, and, sometimes, emotional abandonment. If ever there was a formula for hopelessness, surely it is here among the sixty million AIDS patients in the world today. No wonder so many of them are simply overwhelmed.

I had a friend named Tim who died recently of AIDS. He was by no means the first person I knew who died from AIDS-related causes — is there anybody out there still untouched by this epidemic? — but he was the first I saw die close-up. In slow motion. When he learned he was HIV positive, Tim moved back to Atlanta to be near his family in Alabama. We joked about how we had something in common — death sentences. I told him how I had escaped mine for almost a decade and he seemed to take some encouragement from that. Then, only a year after I met him — when he still showed no signs of his illness — he tried to kill himself. Afterward, when I asked him why, he said he didn't want his family and friends to witness his slow and inevitable death.

For the next year, his parents and I and all his friends waged war on that word "inevitable." His doctors labored heroically to keep him out of the hospital and, for the most part, succeeded. For someone with a T-cell count hovering in the teens, he lived a remarkably normal life. When KS finally made its ugly appearance — on his face — we all worried about his spirits. Fortunately, by then, chemotherapeutic agents were available to keep the lesions under control. With a program of chemotherapy (and a little makeup), he was soon back to normal living again.

Then came the second suicide attempt. The doctors who pumped his stomach said he had taken enough painkillers, sedatives, and antidepressants to kill three people, but all he did was sleep for a long time. Here was proof, I told him when he woke up, that different people respond differently to the same drugs. If he was as lucky with chemotherapy and antivirals as he was unlucky with sleeping pills, he could live long enough to see a cure — or at least the next generation of treatments. I asked his doctor why he would try suicide again just when, thanks to the chemotherapy, his prospects were looking brighter, not dimmer. "Depressed people don't usually commit suicide when they're at the bottom," he said. "It's usually when they're coming up out of a depression and all they see ahead is more of the same. It isn't the depression that kills them, it's the hopelessness."

The last year of Tim's life was one long depression punctuated by repeated trips to the hospital for exotic pneumonias, long periods of intubation, feeding tubes, IV antibiotics, and heavy steroids. When his white blood cell count dropped, he started missing chemo treatments and the KS leapt into the breach. It spread over his face, into his mouth, and down his throat. His body withered away, his liver faltered. At the end, a strange gray mass appeared in his brain. The doctors never had time to find out what it was. In the last real conversation I had with him, he talked about "the tangerine in my head" and how, now, we really did have something in common.

A week before the end, he tried suicide one last time. Only by now he was too weak to make it stick. He just ended up in the hospital again, for the last time, his breathing as frail and shallow as hummingbirds' wings, his skin as yellow as old ivory. "He couldn't find hope anywhere," one of his doctors told me after the end finally came. "Not in his friends, not in his family, and not in us. Everywhere he looked, all he saw was hopelessness."

That he was wrong is only one small tragedy in the panoramic tragedy of AIDS.

In fact, as with cancer, there *are* early signs of hope in the treatment of AIDS — further off and fainter than those for cancer — but hope still. "We are in AIDS where we were in cancer many years ago," says Dr. Pizzo. "There is hope. There's always hope. Many childhood cancers are nearly curable now that were fatal twenty-five years ago. I just don't want to wait twenty-five years for that to happen for pediatric AIDS." On the medical side,

Pizzo and others find hope in the constant development of new agents, like protease inhibitors, to better control the disease and manage its devastating effects, as well as "tremendous advances in the understanding of the biology of the disease." Recently, that better understanding has led to the development of the so-called AIDS cocktail, a combination of drugs that wages a multifront war on the virus, reducing it in some patients to undetectable levels. "People used to be living only two or three years with this disease," says Pizzo. "Now they're living five or ten years. And it can only get better."

That may be only marginal, but hope is a creature of the margins.

What does Pizzo tell his patients, children dying from AIDS with their parents and siblings gathered around their bedsides, many of whom are also infected with the disease? "I say, 'We don't have a cure for this disease today, but we do have things that will buy time,'" says Pizzo, "'and we have to hope together that in buying time, better things are going to become available, and that it's critical that you maintain that hope.'" And how does Pizzo maintain *his* hope in the midst of so much hopelessness? "My job is to continue to look to the future," he says. "Because the battle has to be won in the long run, and it's only going to be won if we keep our hands on the wheel and keep struggling against the odds to get to the next step."

The other doctors I spoke to shared Pizzo's hopefulness. "They thought they couldn't beat polio," says Marston Linehan, "and they did. They thought we couldn't beat cancer, and we are in the process of doing just that. The only way to get there is to keep pressing ahead, and if we do, we will."

On the human side, too, there is reason for hope. Dr. White reports that fewer and fewer of her patients now have to face the disease without the support of their families. "As the disease has become much better known, it is much more accepted and people do turn to their families and their friends," says White. "I don't see patients alone much anymore, and that may be the best thing that could happen to them, short of a cure."

Another "opening" for hope: AIDS, like cancer, has shown great variability from one patient to the next. As I tried so often to tell Tim, AIDS treatments, like cancer treatments, can have a wide range of effects depending on the patient. "We tell people they can always hope that they are going to be among the very good responders to therapy," says Dr. Henry Masur. Some AIDS patients, in fact, have lived long past their death sentences. Whether that's the result of variations in individual immune systems or variations between strains of the AIDS virus isn't known yet, but it is cause for hope. "Whether it's HIV or cancer, or anything else," says Masur, "it's *always* reasonable to be hopeful."

Dr. Klagsbrun, the psychiatrist, finds cause for hope in the fact that some AIDS patients seem to be able to affect, within limits, the progress of their disease. "I've seen enough clinical evidence to support that notion even in the AIDS cases. People who are doing something with their lives seem to hang in longer." He cites the case of a patient of his, a well-known writer. "I've followed him for many years," says Klagsbrun, "and his T-cells seem literally to fluctuate based on whether he's depressed or upbeat. When he feels he's in charge, his life is moving ahead, he's writing, he's being productive, he hardly has time to pay attention to his disease, and his T-cells rise to three or four hundred, when they've been down to two."

Dr. Cimino, at Calvary Hospital, thinks that AIDS is following in cancer's footsteps in another important way. "As with cancer," says Cimino, "we are already working our way toward a view of HIV as a *chronic* disease, not a terminal one. Indeed, people who work with AIDS patients, like Dr. White, have already noted changes in the way those patients think about AIDS. "People now know, at the time of diagnosis, that being HIV positive doesn't mean they're going to die next week," says White. "Because medicine can treat many of the infections that come with AIDS, and because the new drugs can prolong life, many patients no longer think of the disease as an immediate death sentence. They feel that they have some time. That there is something to hope for.

"They know it's going to be a fight to handle these various infections that come up, as well as the side effects of all the drugs they have to take, but most of the HIV patients that I work with want to be a part of that fight. They get quite active and knowledgeable about their disease. That doesn't mean they don't get discouraged sometimes. And because they're more knowledgeable, they know when they're reaching the end of the natural history of their disease, and at that point, they may make a decision not to have certain interventions. But that decision is not a negative thing. It comes not out of total despair but out of a desire to control their illness and their destiny."

Where there is control, there is hope.

"They're giving up but it's not really a giving up," says White. "As with many chronic diseases like cancer, it's a wearing out. They fought the battle, and now they're making a decision: 'This I will do, but this I will not do. I will not go this other step.' This is a triumph over fear, and a major step toward what every patient hopes for and should have, namely dignity."

Where there is dignity, there is hope.

And what about John Grout, the "hopeless" case and desperate cure that began this chapter? Grout didn't have AIDS. He had amyloidosis, a degenerative nerve disease much like Lou Gehrig's disease. It's an inherited malady. Grout's father died of it. The only thing that amyloidosis has in common with AIDS is that it is incurable and fatal. Or, perhaps, was.

Unsatisfied with all the conventional answers, John Grout offered himself up as an experiment. He would be the first person ever to have an "immune system transplant," receiving both the liver and the bone marrow of a donor at the same time. In fact, he virtually invented the experiment. He found the scientist who had done experimental work in immune system transplants (in mice and rats), he convinced the University of Chicago, where he was in line for a liver transplant, to harvest the marrow from his donor. "They pointed out all the reasons it wouldn't work," Grout recalls, "and all the things that were wrong with my argument." But Grout persisted. "This wasn't a dress rehearsal," he says. "You only get one shot."

When he first contacted Dr. Nancy Ascher, the eminent transplant surgeon at the University of California, San Francisco Medical Center, Ascher was wary. "She not only had doubts about whether it would work," Grout recalls, "but she thought it would be irresponsible to do it because they had never tried it first with any animal models." But Grout flew to San Francisco and persuaded Ascher he understood the risks and accepted them. "I knew if I didn't go for it," he says, "I'd regret it for the rest of my life." Grout and his wife rented an apartment in San Francisco, and on September 3, 1994, Dr. Ascher performed the transplant.

Of course, it's been only three years since Grout received a new immune system. Ascher would be the first to say that it's far too early to draw any conclusions.

But not too early to hope.

And what a hope. If the procedure proves successful, it could mean a cure, complete or partial, for all kinds of autoimmune diseases: diabetes (where one out of six health care dollars is spent), severe rheumatoid arthritis, multiple sclerosis, muscular dystrophy.

And AIDS.

Whether or not John Grout survives to old age, though, whether or not this groundbreaking transplant procedure can be used to cure other chronic, "incurable" immune diseases like MS or AIDS, whether or not this is the first step in that direction; *there will be a first step.* Whether or not John Grout is the one, there will be a first. There is always a first. Just as there will be a first AIDS patient cured. Someday, someone will make that miracle happen.

TWENTY-THREE

Doing Fine

PEOPLE ASK ME HOW I'm doing, and depending on who they are, how much time I have, and what I think they really want to know, I give them either the long answer or the short answer. The short answer, of course, is "fine." That's not really wrong. I do consider myself fine — in a day-to-day, nonhistorical sense. Most days I feel fine, I look OK, and except for the multitude of pills and three shots I self-inflict every day, my life isn't that different from any other man in his mid-forties. Of course, I tire more easily than I used to, don't always sleep through the night, etc. Nothing un- usual — unfine — in that.

The long answer includes all of the above, plus a description of how I return every six months to the green hills of Charlottesville for a week-long checkup that involves much poking and prod- ding, scanning and screening, twenty-four-hour this and every- eight-hours that. I may be "still here," but, five years after surgery, so is the tumor — although by best estimates it hasn't grown any in that time. Definitive proof that Dr. Vance's wonder hormone is responsible, however, is hard to come by. Would the tumor have grown without the experimental drug? Would it resume growing if I stopped my thrice-daily injections? I don't know. I don't want to find out. Recent studies show that somatostatin dramatically inhibits angiogenesis, the growth of blood vessels like the ones that make up most of my tumor. In the absence of something better, that's good enough for me.

Every now and then, however, the tumor does make its presence known. The déjà vu spells continued until only recently, waxing and waning from one a day to as many as four. I started keeping a diary to see if I could relate their comings and goings to anything in my life: stress, deadlines, travel, late nights, bad weather, too little (or too much) laughter. The neurologists at U.V.A. dispelled my worst fears: that they were signs that the tumor was "on the move" again. "Just the aftereffects of the surgery," they said: eccentric electrical discharges across the war-torn part of my brain that had suffered through two craniotomies, to say nothing of dozens of bursts of flaming dye and bombardments of radiation.

Then, in 1995, on another Christmas nine years after that fateful one, the spells disappeared. They didn't taper off — fewer each day and then on fewer days — they just stopped, and never returned. So far, at least. For all of medicine's revelations and explanations, the human body remains wondrous strange. I cling to the belief that whatever can go inexplicably wrong can also go inexplicably right.

Actually, "cling" is too strong. The tumor may still be here, but the fear is definitely gone. And that, ultimately, is the more important cure. I no longer lie awake at night, my imagination a boulder of paranoia hurtling through ever bleaker, ever more remote landscapes of possibilities. I no longer wake up dreading that first look in the mirror, that first sip of water, or the first spoken word booby-trapped with one of those long-dreaded explosive consonants. For a long time, I would wake up and before even getting out of bed, run through a series of puckers and burblings and word plays (Peter Piper, etc.), testing my systems like an astronaut on his way to the moon. Every morning.

But not anymore. I no longer even have those slow-motion, Kodak dreams in which I'm running through meadows and jumping over fences the way I could (but seldom did) in my former life, before all this happened. How many forty-five-year-olds still run and jump anyway? The burden of self-pity, as well as the burden of fear — both of which made it hard to enjoy even the best moments of the last decade — have finally been lifted.

What's left in their place is the most unlikely feeling of all — the very last thing I ever expected to feel again — serenity. Freedom from desperation. First, the serenity of knowing that there will be no more Christmas surprises. That's why I spend a week at the U.V.A. hospital twice a year. I've learned the hard way the cost of ignoring or minimizing medical problems. People who live in denial don't realize that they're not avoiding anguish, they're just deferring it — usually to a time when it's too late to do much about it. Then there's the serenity of knowing that if something does happen, if during one of these hospital stays, the doctors do find something — a new tumor or a newly aggressive old one — that it isn't because I dropped the ball. If the worst happens — and it can at any minute, with the help of a drunk driver or a wind shear instead of a tumor — I've made the most of what I had to work with.

And another feeling as well. As I write these final paragraphs, I am sitting upright in a hospital bed on the eighth floor of the big aluminum-clad hospital at the foot of Jefferson's acropolis. The eight-year-old girl in the room next to me suffers violent epileptic seizures. She can't leave her bed without wearing a contraption that looks like a cross between a football player's helmet and a hockey goalie's mask. Every morning, an old man is wheeled by my door by his attentive son and cautiously trailing grandchildren. He is only sixty — fifteen years older than me — but pale and frail as paper. He reminds me of Tim.

And I feel lucky.

I have come back to where I started: feeling lucky. Lucky with my family, lucky with opportunities, lucky with friends, lucky with Steve, and, now, lucky with life. The trick, of course, is to make the most of that luck. Shakespeare was right: Ripeness is all.

That's the long answer.

But "fine" will do.

Index